Type 4 Diabetes

Elevated Insulin. Lower Blood Sugar. 24/7 Pain.

Bob Ranson

BBGmedia

R e s t o n ,   V A

Type 4 Diabetes: Elevated Insulin. Lower Blood Sugar & 24/7 Pain

Copyright © 2007 Robert H. Ranson

All rights reserved.

Published by BBGmedia
1609-B Washington Plaza
Reston, VA 20190
www.bbgmedia.com

First printing in the United States of America
Lulu.com

ISBN: 978-0-6151-3761-2

Designed by Kate Ranson-Walsh
Set in Adobe Garamond Pro and Gil Sans

While the author has made every effort to provide accurate Internet addresses at the time of publication, neither the author nor the publisher assumes any responsibility for errors, or changes that occur after publication. Please refer to www.type4diabetes.com for updated addresses and additional links.

The author may be reached via email: bob@type4diabetes.org

Dedication

To my post-nuclear family of incredibles for loving me so much and pushing me beyond despair, beyond acceptance of the status quo and beyond giving in. With all my love to James, Kate, Brendan, Margee and Geoff.

A Note of Caution

This book is not meant as a replacement for the advice and medical care of your physician. Nor is this book meant to discourage or dissuade you from seeking that advice and care. Diabetes, neuropathy, Alzheimer's and hypoglycemia are serious, potentially fatal, diseases and disorders regardless of the definition used. Consult with your physician on a regular basis if you think you have or have been diagnosed with one or more of these conditions. Do not alter your treatment plan — especially changing or stopping medications — without checking with your doctor. If you have any questions about the content of this book, please consult with your medical advisers.

Acknowledgments

I owe so much to so many for my journey — from cardiac arrest to the amazing discovery that gave me a second life and led to the publication of this book.

While undergoing a routine diagnostic blood pressure test in the fall of 1999, my heart stopped beating. I flatlined. Brought back by a skilled medical team who inserted a pacemaker, I left the hospital with a diagnosis of autonomic neuropathy — a disease that impairs the ability of the heart, digestive system, sexual and other organs to function properly.

Pain, constant pain. Chronic fatigue. Inability to concentrate. Nausea. Sudden, violent diarrhea. All became my constant companions and sapped my enjoyment of life.

But, today I am completely free of pain, related symptoms and the need to take more than a dozen partially-effective daily pills and injections.

What my doctors didn't know I had to learn on my own. My misery was not a direct result of the neuropathy, but due to low blood glucose levels. Simply by raising and maintaining my blood sugar at a level above any recommended by physicians — especially since I had already been diagnosed with diabetes — I earned for myself a great, pain-free, medication-free second life.

I have conquered the pain of neuropathy and I have controlled my "roller-coaster" ride of blood glucose levels through a simple, effective and inexpensive treatment.

What I learned, how I learned it and what it all may mean to millions are the reasons I wrote this book.

So, thanks to Dr. Margaret May Walsh for being such an outstanding editor and life-time supporter, and to Dr. Christopher Bartlett for his medical oversight and review.

Thanks to Kate Ranson-Walsh (www.paperwarp.com) for her "insanely great" design, photography and blogging/website expertise, and to Brendan Ranson-Walsh (www.brendanranson-walsh.com) for the artistic tips and suggestions.

A hearty pat on the back and enormous thanks to James and Geoff Smith for the breakthrough concept of BodyByGeoff Health & Fitness (www.bodybygeoff.com) that pushed me back into shape. Their unique ideas on wellness will spread across the country in short order. And, thanks to their staff of trainers and therapists for taking care of this aging body.

A smile of thanks to Dr. Internal, Dr. Syncope and Dr. Endo for the outstanding medical care over these many years — and for the patience in dealing with a first-class obsessive patient. I have chosen not to use their real names — obviously — out of respect for their privacy. Taken out of context, many of my comments in this book could be misinterpreted as criticism of their medical skills and treatment recommendations. If readers do so, that is a mistake. These skilled physicians have literally saved my life on more than one occasion. If they wish to come forward it will be of each one's own choosing.

Also, a very generous "thank you" to Elaine Shaver for consistently insightful and supportive therapy.

And, not the least, so many thanks to Jerry Newberry, a great friend and supporter who has always been there when I needed him most.

Contents

Quick Glossary

Additional definitions and links are available at
www.type4diabetes.com

Adrenaline: the hormone that helps your body respond to physical or
mental stress. In medical texts the hormone is more often labeled as
epinephrine. Alternative spelling: adrenalin.

Alzheimer's Disease: the most common form of dementia (memory loss
and impaired reasoning) among older people. It involves parts of
the brain that control thought, memory and language.

Disease: a disorder of the function in a human that produces a specific set
of symptoms. Compare with **Syndrome**: a group of symptoms that
are consistently seen together but is not yet recognized as a disease.

Fibromyalgia: a chronic illness of pain (muscle, bone and/or joint), fatigue,
heightened sensitivity to touch and other complications.

Glucose: A simple sugar that serves as a principal source of energy for the
human body.

Hyperglycemia: an excess of blood sugar (glucose) level often associated
with diabetes mellitus (commonly referred to simply as diabetes).

Hypoglycemia: an insufficient level of blood sugar (glucose) to support
normal body functions.

Insulin: a hormone that controls carbohydrate metabolism.

Neuropathy: an abnormal and usually degenerative state of the nervous
system or nerves. The most common forms are autonomic (affect-

ing the involuntary nerves that control your body systems) and peripheral (commonly used to describe sensory problems in hands and feet).

Type 1 Diabetes: autoimmune destruction of insulin-producing cells in the pancreas leasing to hyperglycemia (excess blood sugar)

Type 2 Diabetes: insufficient levels of insulin and/or insulin resistance in cells leading to hyperglycemia. This type accounts for 90-95% of diabetes cases.

Type 3 Diabetes: depletion of insulin in the brain leading to Alzheimer's Disease. New term proposed by a research team at Brown Medical School.

Type 4 Diabetes: elevated insulin levels leading to hypoglycemia (low blood sugar), chronic pain and other neuropathy complications. New term proposed by the author.

Type 4 Diabetes

Introduction

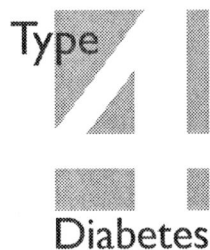

Introduction

Neuropathy. Diabetes. Hypoglycemia. Three different disorders, diseases or syndromes? Or, three different faces on one complex blood sugar problem? A faulty glucose metabolism disease that inflicts severe pain and life-altering discomforts on millions?

As a patient, not a doctor, I find neuropathy, diabetes and hypoglycemia oddly simple and yet mystifyingly complex. Simple in what the terms stand for — having been a graduate college student and adjunct professor long enough to break down words:

■ Neuropathy: nerve + disease

■ Hypoglycemia: low + blood sugar

■ Diabetes Mellitus (formal name and a bit more complex): pass through + sweet

Complex in that we really don't know how they work, how to cure them or even to understand the intricate relationships involved in the progression of these diseases.

My frustrations with neuropathy, diabetes and hypoglycemia put me squarely in a large crowd of patients and physicians. But, I now stand alone — or at least in an extremely small group — in believing that these terms are just three different names for the same complicated disease.

Start with the fact that combinations of these terms already populate medical knowledge:

■ Diabetes + neuropathy: a majority of people with diabetes develop peripheral neuropathy and increasing numbers autonomic neuropathy as well.

■ Diabetes + hypoglycemia: excessive amounts of injected insulin and/or oral diabetes medications leads to hypoglycemia.

The focus of this book centers around this formula for the new term of Type 4 Diabetes:

Type 4 Diabetes = the high glucose complications of diabetes **+** the low glucose complications of hypoglycemia **+** the complications of autonomic neuropathy

This leads to the following set of definitions:

Type 1 autoimmune destruction of insulin-producing cells leading to hyperglycemia (high blood glucose)

Type 2 insulin resistance leading to hyperglycemia (high blood glucose)

Type 3 depletion of insulin in the brain leading to Alzheimer's Disease. *(Please go to Chapter 6 for details)*

Type 4 elevated insulin levels leading to hypoglycemia (low blood glucose), chronic pain and
related complications

In addition, I offer for consideration the following points:

1. The sharp rise of diagnosed cases of autonomic neuropathy attributed to diabetes
   since the early 1990s may be, in fact, due
   to aggressive treatment of diabetes rather
   than the disease itself. With the advent of
   "designer" insulin and a broad spectrum
   of oral Type 2 medications in the 1980s,
   physicians have had the tools to effectively
   drive down the glucose levels of most
   patients.

2. For the past two decades, all too many
   doctors have dismissed hypoglycemia as a
   fake or fad disease. Outside of blood sugar
   levels induced by insulin or oral medications, these physicians claim that hypoglycemia can't possibly exist. Many of these
   claims are based on research studies in the
   1970s using glucose tolerance tests – pro-
   cedures that are now called into question
   by numerous leading diabetes specialists.

3. An aberrant reaction of insulin with
   adrenaline (epinephrine) may play a significant role in the relationship between
   the symptoms of autonomic neuropathy,
   diabetes and hypoglycemia (and perhaps
   even fibromyalgia) seen in many people;
   symptoms of Type 4 Diabetes.

Controversial? Of course.

Without question this book will give rise to another triad: the dismissers, the detractors and the defamers.

I welcome them.

Not that I enjoy being criticized and mocked; I don't. And, yes, being well versed in the principle that 'controversy sells' will cushion some of the barbs. But, selling lots of books is not a goal in and out itself. Rather, I fervently hope a swelling discussion will incite patients to ask their doctors who will then prompt their colleagues in research centers and pharmaceutical companies to spend the time and money for detailed examinations into the concept of Type 4 Diabetes.

I invite the doubt and skepticism, condemnations and derision simply because the more people say about this topic the more my mission advances. I suffered for many years; others are suffering even worse with little or no hope. The future will bring misery to countless more people. Why? My mission is simple: to bring as much of this misery for others to an end.

I am many things, but unique is not one of them. I discovered a fundamental link between my pain, neuropathy, low glucose and diabetes. Through this discovery I developed a simple, inexpensive and extremely effective treatment to all but eliminate the pain and litany of unpleasantness. If this treatment works for me surely it must as well for how many others? Hundreds, thousands, millions?

As more and more people ask the same questions, others will be inclined to spend the time and money to find the answers, to tell us who can benefit and why, and what are the long term prospects for those that choose this path.

This book narrates a personal journey; my journey through the limitations of understanding and treating the broad spectrum of glucose metabolism disorders that are the scourge of our society and times.

Accepting the rather presumptuous nature of this book – that a patient takes upon himself to correct medical misunderstandings and redefine medical terminology – I compound that further by believing that this work falls within the category of good literature by posing more questions than it answers.

My journey through "Type 4 Diabetes" does offer several important answers, clues to many more and poses a great deal of questions for others to consider. Through this I offer a potential for the treatment that could save tens of thousands, perhaps millions of people from constant pain and suffering.

The treatment I use and suggest in this book works for me. BUT, THAT DOES NOT MEAN IT WILL WORK FOR YOU. I hope that it will help, but the *consequences could be severe if it doesn't*. So, DO NOT accept this as a treatment prescription for you without first consulting with your doctor — especially if you have diabetes. Yes, it is true, as you will read, that I ignored the learned expertise and recommendations of my doctors and went in my own direction. However, I ALWAYS KEPT THEM INFORMED – just in case.

HOW SHOULD YOU READ THIS BOOK?

You could, of course, read the book from cover to cover. Let me, though, offer a guide to understanding its structure and alternative ways to reading this work.

- Each of the first 10 chapters begins with a step I journey from cardiac arrest in 1999 to a new life free of pain and misery in 2006. For those of you with an understanding of neuropathy, diabetes and hypoglycemia, you may choose to just read "The Journey" portions of each chapter. Each page of "The Journey" is framed with a gray border to reinforce the nature of these sections being a diary.

- At the end of "The Journey" segment in

each chapter you'll find a section entitled "In Detail." In those sections, I offer insight into the current understanding of the elements that constitute Type 4 Diabetes. As subjective as "The Journey" segments are, I strive for objective in the "In Detail" portions.

■ Each "In Detail" section provides you with an understanding of my own research, step by step, in developing the concept of Type 4 Diabetes. I am only presenting enough information to help those unfamiliar with the terms to gain valuable insight. The sections are not a replacement for the many well-written books and resources available for patients suffering from these disorders as well as their caregivers. And, the "In Detail" sections certainly are not meant to constitute a formal research paper on a medical topic. I am providing a launching point upon which more capable others can write in depth.

■ In most chapters, you will also discover "In Addition" segments. Here, you will find links to printed and Internet-based resources that can assist you in learning more about a particular topic.

■ My concluding chapter and appendices summarize my principle arguments and makes the case for the concept of Type 4 Diabetes. The experts among you may be tempted to read this introduction and then skip to the conclusion. Fine. But, if you remain a skeptic at the end, please take the time to read "The Journey" for an understanding of where I have been and the perspective from which I make these arguments.

WHO SHOULD READ THIS BOOK?

Please take the time to read this book if you have:

- Diabetes and are concerned about neuropathy

- Neuropathy and are worried about the potential for developing Type 2 Diabetes

- Hypoglycemia or experienced the symptoms of low blood sugar (alone or as a part of fibromyalgia) and have been told "it's all in your head"

- A concern that you or a loved one could have diabetes, neuropathy and/or low blood sugar.

- A belief that patients should be more responsible for their own medical treatments.

IS THIS A "BOOK", "BLOOK" OR A "WEB BOOK"?

Actually, it's all three.

Book. Traditional, printed and self-contained.

Blook. New term for a book based on a "blog" (a website where entries are written in a journal style), or for book contents serialized on a blog. Indeed, content from this book appears in chapter form on the related website: www.Type4Diabetes.org

    WebBook. A newer term for a book integrated with a web site and based on research primarily obtained from web sources available to all. Most of the endnotes and reference citations found in this book will lead you to sites on the web that you can view. I chose that path intentionally. I want readers, skeptics or supporters, to have the ability to easily check out my citations and read more of the same. I also make use of the *Wikipedia*, the free online encyclopedia. I find great value in this incredible tool and have found it to be as accurate, if not more so, than many other "traditional" reference sources.

    Many scholars will question this web-based research model. But, I think it wise as well as instructive. The Internet ranks, along with the Gutenberg press, as the leading inventions of the last 1,000 years. The ability to access nearly the entire compendium of human knowledge with a few keystrokes from anywhere in the world staggers most minds. My quest is to encourage discussion about this topic and to further research by professionals as well as patients. I offer my links as additional tools in your search.

    The integration of a traditional book and a website eliminates the most frustrating aspect of printed materials. They are often out of date the moment they are printed. I, too, had to close off my journey at a specific point even as I continue to learn more, to acquire more and understand more each day. What occurred after the last word was written in this book can be found on the website: **www.Type4Diabetes.org**. I invite you to visit the site, read more and contribute your own ideas, thoughts and experiences in the Type 4 Diabetes blog.

    Our journey together has only begun.

Thank you.　　　　　*December 2006*

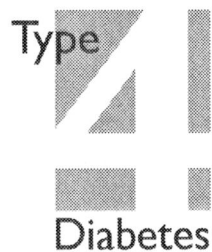

Type
Diabetes

Chapter I

- The Beginning

- Tilt-Table Test

- Pacemaker

Chapter 1
The Journey Begins

I am not a doctor. I am a patient. And this is my journey.

While undergoing a routine diagnostic blood pressure test in 1999, I went into complete cardiac arrest. Less than 10 minutes into a standard "tilt-table test" to diagnose blood pressure problems, my heart stopped. The last thing I remembered was the alarming sound of cardiac monitors indicating a flatline — along with a flood of sensations that is best described as the worst experience in my life.

Perhaps a fitting metaphor for this entire journey, those moments of misery ended in a flash of darkness followed by brilliance and then a truly wonderful period of euphoria — a brief journey to the next life . Leaving aside lessons learned from the moments in the light to be revisited over and over again, I became aware of my doctors and nurses yelling at me to breathe.

"Now, that's a stupid thing to say," I thought, as the light receded and my other senses returned to an active state. "Why would anyone have to ask you to breathe?" We do that automatically, don't we? Yes, but when the "automatic system" fails, there is a "manual backup "that only works when you try. Welcome to a new world!

I suddenly had to cope with autonomic neuropathy, a disease of the central nervous system that can adversely impact every organ in your body. Essentially, your nerves don't transmit the correct information — or any information at all — from the brain to a body part. Most of us can handle irregular signals to our stomach or intestines, or even no signal for a few minutes here and there. It's when your body attempts that trick with your heart that life appears in sharp focus.

Thankfully, I had some very bright doctors who suspected something serious before I climbed onto the table and prepared for the worst. They were right and literally saved my life. Brought back by a skilled medical team who later inserted a pacemaker, I began my journey — painful, frustrating and expensive — into the worst and best of American health care in the opening years of the 21st century.

Without any detailed warnings about what might happen during the tilt-table test, I couldn't cope with the abrupt decision to "sign the paper" and let the doctors insert a pacemaker into my chest ASAP. Ask me then what I knew about those little devices and my response would have been, "Ah, they're for old people with heart problems." Not a very educated response.

And, not being a shy or unquestioning patient (an understatement given the nature of this book!), I punted and begged off for the time being until I could talk it over with my partner who had just flown in on a West Coast red-eye flight. James had arrived in time to pick me up at home, drop me off at the hospital for the early morning procedure and then return to a state of much needed sleep, confident that he had about five hours of quiet before picking me up from the medical facility.

Kicked awake after only 90 minutes with the numbing message that "We need you at the hospital immediately; there has been a problem during his test," James was as little prepared mentally as I was for making any decisions — let alone something as serious as a pacemaker. And, more importantly, neither of us had any basis for understanding the reasons why a pacemaker would be necessary.

What is the right decision to make at a moment such as this? I had no idea then nor do I now. We opted for punting again and checked out of the hospital as soon as possible to "sleep on it." As if we could sleep.

For hours we sat over cups of coffee reviewing the events that had led to this crucial decision point.

I was a Type A personality in my late 40s. In my role as the head of the public relations group for a major American advertising agency my working life consisted of helping large clients get out and stay out of image problems. Adrenaline was my juice and stress my partner. As such, it didn't seem much of a stretch that I started experiencing what appeared to be blood pressure problems at both work and the occasional moments of play.

The first I became aware of anything out of line were brief moments of dizziness after a sudden movement or standing in one place for a long period of time. It struck me as odd when I had the sensation of losing a second or two of time. Then I dropped coffee mugs once at work and once washing dishes at home after standing up suddenly. With a sheepish smile, I just told all those that noticed, "Sorry, just clumsy today." Right.

The growing worry peaked after 30 minutes of lap swimming one day. Not a hard swim, but I felt very tired and "odd" as I walked into the locker room. The next thing I remember was looking up at the ceiling from the floor with no idea how I landed on my back. Perhaps a visit to the doctor would be in order.

In the days leading up to that eventful visit, I spent lots of time reviewing my own medical history as best I could remember. Growing up in a medical household taught some lessons well. My dad ran a hospital and my mother excelled as a psychiatric nurse and later as a public school nurse back in the days. I had the privilege of outstanding medical care on demand and had grown accustomed to it early. I believed from the start that the best medical care occurs when patients provide their doctors with meaningful insights and clear summaries of issues. It is part of the training.

In preparing my mental notes for the doctor's briefing, I recalled a series of incidents in my junior high school days when I had experienced similar symptoms and brief fainting spells. After rounds of tests, my parents were told that nothing "spectacular" could be found. Rather the physicians concluded that the stress of adolescence was bringing on transient periods of low blood sugar. The recommended treatment consisted of carrying hard candy and caffeine pills to be taken when "the feelings start."

In retrospect, it was a very relevant diagnosis and treatment approach. Not bad for the days before managed care.

Despite all of my preparation, I entered my internist's office in the summer of 1999 with the typical sense that "Everything will be normal when he sees me. Then I will leave his office, go home and be sick again."

Not this time. Sitting on the exam table, I felt the room begin to spin and the floor appeared mighty close and welcome. Having been my lead physician for 10 years, Dr. Internal knew things were a "tad off" and watched as my blood pressure continued to drop for no apparent reason.

An hour or so of observations and discussions ensued with my doctor growing increasingly perplexed and obviously concerned. I considered my doctor to be the best medical diagnostician. I still do. I knew he wouldn't stop that evening until he had some idea of what was wrong. And he did have an idea.

With a gentle start he left his office and then returned with a sense of direction. "I'm not quite sure. But, I just read an article a few weeks back written by a specialist in cardiovascular issues about new evidence of blood pressure irregularities." He went on to note, "I have never seen any patients that fit his description until now. I think you just may be the first to fit the bill."

He declined to provide further information for a variety of reasons, as I later learned. The most prominent in his mind being the avoidance of needless concern and stress at a completely inappropriate time. A wise, very wise decision. At the time, nearly all general practitioners and internists presented with my symptoms would likely have told their patients it was all due to stress and to "exercise more." As a result, untold numbers of men and women in my age group have died from cardiac arrest weeks and months after their fateful visit.

Needless deaths? Yes. Malpractice? No, not at the time.

My doctor acted on the best information at the time and saved my life by nearly carrying me to the cardiologist's office for the tilt-table test. He was right. And he was just as right to call me at home after the tilt-table test and cardiac arrest to warn me in not-so-subtle words that without the pacemaker I could expect to "drop dead someday soon standing in line at the grocery store."

It took two surgeries to properly place a pacemaker in my chest and weeks of calibration to get it "tuned" properly to my body's rhythms.

These doctors, and others who came into my life, were so right about the immediate problem and treatment, but so wrong about the underlying condition and long-term effective treatment.

They just didn't have the information to make better decisions.

In Detail

TILT-TABLE TEST

A tilt-table test is an established medical procedure to help diagnose sudden drops in blood pressure as the underlying cause for symptoms such as fainting spells, dizziness or lightheadedness. In addition to low blood pressure, these same symptoms may be due to low blood sugar or abnormal heart rhythms.

The test is performed on a table that pivots (at the end where your feet rest) from flat to upright (standing position). You are strapped to the table for two reasons: to keep you from falling off, obviously, and to keep you from moving your legs. The reason for keeping your legs constrained is to prevent you from using your large leg muscles to help balance blood pressure.

The rapid drops in your blood pressure may be due to a hyperactive reflex that causes the blood vessels to suddenly dilate (widen). Keeping your leg muscles from "kicking in" allows doctors to more fully understand the nature of your problems.

An adverse reaction on the tilt table could be, as is in my case, the result of a hyperactive reflex that causes the blood vessels to suddenly dilate (widen). Another major reason for an adverse reaction is the inability of the body to quickly regulate blood pressure, especially when you stand up.

The test can last an hour or more, and for many it is just plain boring. The table moves you up and down, lying to standing, as medical technicians monitor your heart rate, blood pressure and other indicators. Sometimes, doctors inject a drug to hasten any adverse reactions.

Since my doctors already suspected an adverse, possibly an extreme, reaction, I was "wired" to the max. A probe had been inserted through an artery in my thigh, monitor patches were attached everywhere, a sonar probe was strapped to my head to track pressure in my head and an intravenous line was inserted in my arm for fluids and medications. Four video cameras watched from every angle along with half a dozen doctors, nurses and technicians.

After 10 minutes of lying still to establish baselines readings, a technician threw the switch sending the table upright. Unfortunately, as the table was swung up, the hospital gown dropped away so the only thoughts going through my brain at the time: "Wonderful. I get to spend the next two hours hanging out in my birthday suit, on camera. Why didn't I start that damn diet sooner?"

You have to think of something.

However, not for for too long in my case. Within minutes a staggering feeling of "unwellness" spread from my chest outward. For me, the time to think about covering back up had passed.

Depending on the severity of the reaction, your doctor may prescribe medications, lifestyle changes and/or a pacemaker. In my case, I ended up with all three.

PACEMAKER

Developed in 1958 by an electrical engineering graduate of Cornell University, Wilson Greatbatch[1], the implantable cardiac pacemaker quickly became a lifesaving medical tool for millions of people. Together with Dr. William Chardack, chief of surgery at the Veterans Administration Hospital in Buffalo, NY, Greatbatch oversaw the first American implant in 1960. He expected that as many as 10,000 devices would eventually be implanted each year. He underestimated. Today, more than 600,000 pacemakers are implanted worldwide each year.

Several companies manufacture pacemakers for implant

in the United States, including Avery Biomedical, Biotronik, Boston Scientific, Sorin Group, St. Jude Medical and Medtronic, the company behind the unit in my chest.

The basic function of a pacemaker is to replace an absent nerve impulse meant to signal the heart to contract, or beat. The pacemaker monitors the heart's electrical activity. When it senses that too long a time has gone by between signals to contract, it fills in the blank. "Too long" is measured in fractions of seconds.

As the sophistication of microcomputer circuitry improves, even as it shrinks, the capabilities of pacemakers steadily improve. Many devices take into account the level of physical activity and alter the beating rhythm.

A distinct variation on the pacemaker is the implantable cardiac defibrillator, such as the one in Vice President Richard Cheney's chest. These units not only sense and provide proper pulsing for heart rhythms, but send an electrical shock to tame a heart that is beating too fast to provide for adequate blood flow.

Surgery to implant a pacemaker is usually done with just local anesthesia and lasts under an hour. There is minimal discomfort during the procedure as the device is inserted under the skin and above the pectoral muscles usually on your left side. Two or more wires are threaded through veins leading to your heart and the ends of the wire are inserted into the heart muscle. You can expect a fair amount of bruising and soreness for the first few weeks, but the discomfort is manageable for the most part.

In my case, the structure of my circulatory system made implanting a device difficult on the left side. The initial procedure lasted more than 2 ½ hours without success. A infection at the surgical site led a second doctor to complete the insertion a day later on my right side. So, I ended up with matching bruises on my chest that resembled a male pec implant gone bad.

Periodically, I have the device checked through a simple procedure where a monitor is placed over the pacemaker and information passed through the skin. There is no discomfort. A doctor downloads an amazing amount of information from the pacemaker. "So I see you were very busy last Thursday night at 2 am. Having fun?"

At first the checkups occurred every few weeks. Now, they occur every six months to a year. That frequency will increase again as I get closer to the end of the battery's life. When it's time for a replacement, a doctor will make a small incision, remove the old unit and put in a new one.

For the time being, my goal is to prolong the life of the unit as much as possible by decreasing the amount of time my pacemaker beats for me. That's a part of the rest of the story.

In Addition

To learn more about the tilt-table test and pacemakers:

■ **Read**

- "Tilt Table Test," Gale Encyclopedia of Medicine by Jeffrey P. Larson RPT, January 1, 2002 <http://amazon.com>.

- Wilson Greatbatch, The Making of the Pacemaker (Amherst, NY: Prometheus Books, 2000

- Blair P. Grubb and Brian Olshansky, ed. Syncope: Mechanisms and Management (Malden, MA: Blackwell Publishing, 2000)

■ **Search:**

- "Cardiac Pacemaker," November 15, 2006 < http://en.wikipedia.org/wiki/Cardiac_pacemaker>.

- "Pacemakers," November 30, 2006 <http://www.american-heart.org/presenter.jhtml?identifier=4676>.

- "Pacemakers," 2005 < http://www.nlm.nih.gov/medlineplus/tutorials/pacemakers/htm/index.htm>.

- "Tilt-Table Test," April 24, 2002 < http://www.medicinenet.com/tilt-table_test/article.htm>.

- "Tilt-Table Test," September 23, 2006 < http://en.wikipedia.org/wiki/Tilt_table_test>.

■ Endnotes

1. Wilson Greatbatch, <u>The Making of the Pacemaker</u> (Amherst, NY: Prometheus Books, 2000

You can locate updated information
and additional links by visiting:
www.type4diabetes.com.

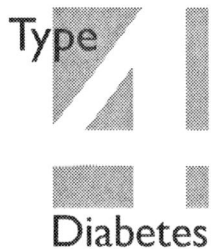
Type
Diabetes

Chapter 2

- ■ Neuropathy

- ■ Dysautonomia

Chapter 2
Introduction to Neuropathy

From a patient's perspective, the world of American health care seems as mystifying a blur as reading Tolstoy's *War and Peace*, written in the original Russian language with ample portions of ego, money and politics.

There abound puzzles to solve, mind-numbing codes to break, indecipherable jargon, turf wars that make no sense and a constant barrage of questions - all involving money. Is it covered? Can I afford it? Will someone else pay for it? Why do the drug companies charge so much? Why doesn't the government do something about it?

Everyone's to blame. And everyone, every organization, every institution, every agency firmly believes that it is right.

In the years since 1999, I have debated these questions and so many more. The health care system today is full of wonderful, talented, caring people scrambling to do what is "right." But, with so many rules, concerns and contradictory information it is a near miracle that anyone really gets the help needed.

In the weeks that followed the insertion of the pacemaker into my heart, too many times I sat in the cardiologist's office totally dumbfounded and frustrated, trying to get an answer to the obvious, Why is that $24,000 device in my chest? Way past being satisfied by the "You are going to die" response from Dr. Internal, I needed some information to tell me why I was so sick.

The responses from Dr. Pacemaker always began with "We're not sure, but … " and ended with then meaningless terms such as "neurocardiogenic syncope or orthostatic intolerance dysautonomia or something like that." Oh, well, that clears it all up!

The best responses, after much prodding, were the simplest. We don't really know. We may never know. Your heart isn't getting the proper nerve impulses. Sometimes, for some reason, it doesn't get any nerve impulses.

My insatiable quest for more information began. It hasn't ended.

Through the post-surgery and lots-of-new-drugs fog, some clarity did emerge in the form of textbook definitions. [1]

Syncope. A medical term for fainting.

Neurocardiogenic. A condition that includes sudden loss of consciousness from a change in the function of the autonomic nervous system.

Orthostatic intolerance dysautonomia. An inability to tolerate standing up, due to a sensation of lightheadedness or dizziness.

Coping with this haze of jargon became easier with the realization that the Latin and Greek barrage didn't happen from an attempt to obscure or cover someone's medical butt. Rather, it represented a fundamental lack of real information and sufficient test results to pinpoint an exact cause or long-term diagnosis. Now, that's real frustration.

It took the general acceptance of the tilt-table test in the early 1990s to bring meaningful understanding of the serious problems inherent in autonomic nervous system dysfunction. As noted in the **In Detail** section of the previous chapter, only a small percentage of those who undergo the tilt-table test suffer an extreme heart-related problem. But when we do, the incident is significant. It is a telltale warning to doctors that, for whatever the underlying reason, our autonomic nervous systems are severely impaired.

We need help, whether it be from a pacemaker, daily medications or drastic lifestyle changes. In my case, the recommended treatment consisted of all three.

Unsatisfied with the answers provided by Dr. Pacemaker, I sought assistance from the source: the doctor who authored one of the few books and research papers, at the time, on this entire subject. Far easier said than done, my getting to be his patient took some effort and an expensive plane trip to the research center where he practiced.

The time and money were invested wisely. Aside from being one of the most amazing, gracious, intelligent and charming people ever to have shaken my hand, this doctor stunned me even before a formal introduction. "Before you turn around," he said as he entered the room, "I can tell you that you are naturally blond, have blue eyes and your favorite sport is swimming because it is the only one that gives you a high." Nice parlor trick, I thought.

Not a trick at all; just a demonstration of incredible insights into a genetic malfunction of the nervous system. Be it autonomic neuropathy or autonomic dysautonomia or variants thereof, the genetic abnormalities associated with these conditions convey with the same genes as those that give me the Germanic look of my maternal grandparents: blond hair and blue eyes.

The swimming assumption, the doctor added, comes from the fact that someone with the condition of orthostatic intolerance dysautonomia has problems with maintaining proper blood pressure in the brain while standing upright. Blood tends to pool in the lower portion of the body, primarily the legs, and drain away from the neck up unless you are lying down. That's true in general with humans, but exaggerated in those of us with this nervous malfunction.

Exercising in a prone position (swimming), combined with the pressure of the water on the legs, greatly enhances proper balancing of blood pressure throughout the entire body. Swimming, the only enjoyable exercise for those of us with this condition provides true cardio benefits without over-stressing the body. We enjoy the sensations and the more natural blood flow creates the exercise high.

Already impressing beyond words, Dr. Syncope further dazzled me by comparing me to an astronaut, my childhood fantasy. He told me of a "dirty little secret of NASA" and the fact that we can't go to Mars, no matter what the politicians say, "because our bodies can't make the trip." Aside from a genetic cause and possible viral infections, about the only other way possible to develop autonomic neuropathy requires "being weightless in space for more than six months."

According to the good doctor, the Russians discovered this when several cosmonauts were inadvertently left in space just after the Soviet decline. The Soviets lacked the funds to launch the Soyuz craft on a regular schedule to retrieve the stranded space travelers from the Russian space station, Mir. The returning cosmonauts couldn't walk at first and it wasn't just due to the degeneration of the leg muscles, as was reported. Rather, the cosmonauts fainted due to critical blood pressure problems and irregular heart beats.

Fortunately for these comrades, their version of the disorder is temporary and reversible after months of rest. But, the doctor noted, put a few astronauts on an 8-12 month trip to Mars and sudden fainting spells would just be the beginning of problems upon entering the pull of Martian gravity or, worse, returning to Earth's higher gravity. Astronauts in prolonged weightlessness would have sudden cardiac arrests. Without finding an effective treatment, we just can't go.

"Relax," he told me. "Research money is coming from the government to a few researchers and centers to learn more about these autonomic disorders and how to treat them. You'll just benefit from the mission to Mars!" Beam me up, Scotty!

I felt huge relief knowing that someone really did understand my medical problem. The jargon haze cleared up with the revelation that different researchers were pushing different names for the same set of disorders. This is all about researchers "owning a disease," a concept new to me even though I grew up in a medical family.

What I want to own is a large yacht, an electric car, a vacation home on Cape Cod. A disease? No, thank you. But, then again, I am not a doctor.

Broadly put, doctors want to own a disease, a condition or a treatment for very basic reasons: recognition and research grants. Money is not just the mother's milk of politics; it's the elixir that nourishes the health care community. Stake a claim, get it recognized and research grants from the government, foundations and the pharmaceutical industry come your way. Cause and effect.

To illustrate the point, consider Dr. Syncope. He is a trained and certified cardiologist. He also properly lays claim to being a specialist in electrophysiology, in other words, neurology. He is a specialist in nervous disorders. This is far more than a matter of simple semantics. As one of the pioneers in the field of nervous disorders and their impact on the cardiovascular system, Dr. Syncope is stepping into the playing field claimed by the neurologists, a.k.a., brain doctors. More problematic, he is stepping into the pool of grants available to study neurological conditions.

Intrigued? The next time you are sitting in an emergency room, just ask which specialist handles the body from the waist up and which handles the waist down.

The only consequence of all of this that mattered to me,

as a patient, lay in the confusion over which label to affix to my problem with getting proper nerve signals to my heart and other organs automatically.

While this is perhaps an oversimplification, dysautonomia and related terms tended to get a warmer welcome from the cardiologists/electrophysiologists. Do you prefer autonomic neuropathy? Consider yourself more aligned with the neurologists. It's all Greek (and Latin) to me.

In Detail

In chapter 1, I discussed my adverse tilt table test being the result of a hyperactive reflex suddenly slowing my heart rate. This condition is known as neurocardiogenic syncope. The word comes from a combination of "nervous system" + "heart related" + "fainting".

Another condition that produces an adverse tilt table reaction is neurocardiogenic orthostatic hypotension ("nervous system" + "heart related" + "low blood pressure") or orthostatic intolerance dysautonomia ("standing" + "intolerance" + "malfunction of the autonomic nervous system").

Unfortunately for those of us who are patients, all the medical jargon floating around diseases of the automatic (autonomic) nervous system presents a huge hurdle. Let me attempt to provide additional clarity.

WHAT'S IN A NAME?

Do I have dysautonomia or neuropathy? It depends on whom you ask.

According to the *National Library of Medicine:* [2]

Dysautonomia: a disorder of the autonomic nervous system that causes disturbances in all or some autonomic functions and may result from the course of a disease (as diabetes).

Neuropathy: an abnormal and usually degenerative state of the nervous system or nerves.

Peripheral neuropathy is defined in this database, but not the autonomic form.

In the *Wikipedia*:

Dysautonomia: any disease or malfunction of the autonomic nervous system. This includes postural orthostatic tachycardia syndrome (POTS), neurocardiogenic syncope, mitral valve prolapse dysautonomia, pure autonomic failure, multiple system atrophy (Shy-Drager syndrome), and a number of lesser-known disorders.[3]

Neuropathy: any disease that affects the nervous system. In common usage, however, neuropathy is short for peripheral neuropathy, meaning a disease of the peripheral nervous system, in other words, a disease affecting one or more nerves.[4]

Autonomic neuropathy: a disease of the non-voluntary, non-sensory nervous system (i.e. the Autonomic Nervous System) affecting mostly the internal organs - such as the bladder muscles, the cardiovascular system, the digestive tract, and the genital organs. These nerves are not under a person's conscious control and function automatically. They do not run through the spinal cord. Most commonly, autonomic neuropathy is seen in persons with long-standing diabetes mellitus type 1 and 2.[5]

The World Health Organization's International Classification of Diseases (ICD 10) lists both dysautonomia and neuropathy under the heading of "Diseases of the Nervous System, without distinctive clarification. The ICD 10 links diabetes with peripheral neuropathy and not dysautonomia. To the latter, the ICD 10 links hereditary sensory and autonomic neuropathy. [6]

Go to the website for the National Dysautonomia Research Foundation (NDRF.org) and you will note that the foundation accepts autonomic neuropathy as being a synonym for dysautonomia. Obviously, the terms cry out for some standardization.

In this book, I am using the term **Autonomic Neuropathy** to apply to the disease I have and shorthand for any disease impairment of the autonomic nervous system. To me that makes sense.

DIABETIC NEUROPATHY

The dramatic rise of the past two decades in the number of cases of autonomic neuropathy linked to diabetes is evidenced in the detailed information on the topic supplied by the American Diabetes Association:[7]

Nerves send messages to and from your brain about pain, temperature and touch. They tell your muscles when and how to move. They also control body systems that digest food and pass urine. About half of all people with diabetes have some form of nerve damage. It is more common in those who have had the disease for a number of years. Nerve damage from diabetes is called diabetic neuropathy. It can lead to many kinds of problems.

But if you keep your blood glucose levels on target, you may help prevent or delay nerve damage. There are treatments that can help as well.

What types of nerve damage can occur?

There are two common types of nerve damage. The first is sensorimotor neuropathy, also known as peripheral neuropathy. This can cause tingling, pain, numbness, or weakness in your feet and hands. The second is called autonomic neuropathy. This type can lead to:

- Digestive problems such as feeling full, nausea,

- Vomiting, diarrhea, or constipation

- Problems with how well your bladder works

- Problems having sex

- Dizziness or faintness

- Loss of the typical warning signs of a heart attack

- Loss of the warning signs of low blood glucose

- Increased or decreased sweating

- Changes in how your eyes react to light and dark

In Addition

To learn more about neuropathy:

■ Read

- David S. Goldstein and Linda Joy Smith, <u>The NDRF Handbook for Patients with Dysautonomias</u> (Armonk, NY: Futura Media Services, 2002)

- Norman Latov, <u>Peripheral Neuropathy: When the Numbness, Weakness, and Pain Won't Stop</u>, (Demos Publishing, 2006)

■ Search

- "Autonomic Neuropathy," <u>MayoClinic.com</u>, April 13, 2006, < http://www.mayoclinic.com/health/autonomic-neuropathy/ DS00544>.

- "Recognizing and Treating Diabetic Autonomic Neuropathy," <u>Cleveland Clinic Journal of Medicine</u> by Aaron Vinik and Tomris Erbas, < http://www.ccjm.org/pdffiles/Vinik1101.pdf>

- "Peripheral Neuropathy," <u>MedlinePlus</u>, April 2006, < http:// www.nlm.nih.gov/medlineplus/ency/article/000593.htm>.

■ Visit

- <u>National Dysautonomia Research Foundation</u>, September 2006, < http://ndrf.org/>.

- <u>The Neuropathy Association</u>, 2006, < http://www.neuropathy. org>.

■ Endnotes

1. David Goldsmith and Linda Joy Smith, <u>The NDRF Handbook for Patients with Dysautonomia</u> (Armonk, NY: Futura Media

Services, 2002) 285-309

2. <u>National Library of Medicine</u> < http://www.nlm.nih.gov>.

3. "Dysautonomia." Wikipedia, The Free Encyclopedia. 29 Aug 2006, 00:49 UTC. Wikimedia Foundation, Inc. 1 Dec 2006 <http://en.wikipedia.org/w/index.php?title=Dysautonomia&old id=72509499>.

4. "Neuropathy." Wikipedia, The Free Encyclopedia. 15 Sep 2006, 15:49 UTC. Wikimedia Foundation, Inc. 1 Dec 2006 <http://en.wikipedia.org/w/index.php?title=Neuropathy&oldid=75897 578>.

5. "Autonomic neuropathy." Wikipedia, The Free Encyclopedia. 2 Mar 2006, 22:08 UTC. Wikimedia Foundation, Inc. 1 Dec 2006 <http://en.wikipedia.org/w/index.php?title=Autonomic_n europathy&oldid=41959728>.

6. "International Classification of Diseases," World Health Organization, 2006 < http://www.who.int/classifications/icd/en/>.

7. "Diabetic Neuropathy (Nerve Damage) and Diabetes," American Diabetes Association, December 2006 < http://www.diabetes.org/type-1-diabetes/diabetic-neuropathy.jsp>.

You can locate updated information and links about items listed in this section by visiting: www.type4diabetes.com.

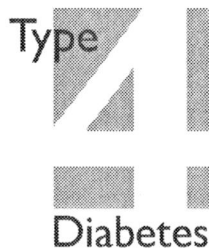

Type
Diabetes

Chapter 3

- Peripheral Neuropathy

- Autonomic Neuropathy

- Medications

- Blood Pressure

- Vasoconstrictor

Chapter 3
Too Much Pain. Too Many Meds.

Regardless of the esteem to which one holds the current pharmaceutical industry, we cannot be complacent about the benefits brought by the hundreds of drugs that touch each of our lives.

Catch a cold? Most of us run to the doctor for something, even if we know that nothing really works on the virus itself. Our response, for better or for worse, is conditioned. We accept the inherent value of the available medications. And, we trust that our doctor prescribes and the pharmacist fulfills the appropriate medication and dosage.

Since I spent 70% of my first grade year home in bed with every possible childhood illness (and a few more than once), you'll get no arguments from me about the merits of drugs. Watching my daughter go through much of the same illnesses at a slightly earlier age only reinforced my faith in pharmaceuticals.

For most of us, drug conditioning extends to reading warning labels about the potentially nasty effects of taking drug A while on medication B. Sometimes we ask for more information, other times we rely on educated guesses based on prior experience. We know that certain drug combinations indeed can be lethal.

The research upon which these warnings are based is a "simple" combination of two drugs. But, what if you take three different prescription drugs at the same time. Four? Five? Or maybe an even dozen?

The "simple" truth? Nobody knows. You are on your own and it is just scary.

Thus my overall anxious mood in the first 12-18 months post the cardiac arrest. In that period, my various doctors placed me on more than 20 different medications, in various combinations and dosages, all in a valued and valiant effort to minimize the impact of autonomic neuropathy. Pain. Legs. Head. 24/7. Nausea. Sudden, violent diarrhea. Constant dizziness. Low blood pressure. High blood pressure. Anxiety.

For most of us with autonomic neuropathy, there just isn't a single wonder drug. For that matter, there isn't an effective cocktail of many medications. At *best*, my drug therapy worked *most* of the time to reduce *some* of the pain. A handful of pills for breakfast, a few more for with lunch, a few more at dinner and then last call at bedtime. Not just oral medications were required. To get a handle on the worst of the pain, I could count on injecting myself with a vasoconstrictor medication 2-3x a week. Try that if you hate needles or have a blinding headache.

With autonomic neuropathy, we frequently suffer from uncontrollable pain in our legs due, in part, to the constant and erroneous effort on the part of our circulatory system to lower blood pressure by dilating the vessels in the lower part of our body. After a while, that swelling hurts. Badly.

A vasoconstrictor such as contained in many migraine treatments helps by shrinking the vessels and removing the pressure on surrounding tissues. Caffeine is also a vasoconstrictor and is a key ingredient in over the counter (OTC) medications such as Excedrin Migraine (along with aspirin and acetaminophen). Carefully taken, caffeine can be of help, but may bring along unwelcome side-effects as a stimulant.

Over time, I developed my own pain scale based on the severity and speed with which the pain came on. A low level meant 500 mgs of Bufferin and Tylenol. Moderate attack of pain called for a tablet of Frova. "Lord have mercy!" demanded an injection of Imitrex. And, all of this occurred several times week even as I swallowed other pain medications such as 600 mgs of Neurontin (commonly prescribed for chronic pain) on a daily basis.

Fortunately, and unfortunately, I knew that I was not alone in this agony. Little more than two years after my diagnoses, a friend of many years also came down with autonomic neuropathy. His pain quickly became worse and passed 800 mgs of Neurontin in a flash. Unable to control the pain, as of this writing, he manages each day with large doses of morphine. It is not a nice way to live.

Prior to diabetes entering my life, I had little exposure to or knowledge of the related neuropathy labeled as peripheral since it impacts the extremities of the body: hands and feet. For people with diabetes, peripheral neuropathy has been and continues to be of major concern. The loss of proper nerve function in the hands and feet is the most common cause of amputations.

The relation of these two disorders to each other remains clouded in much conjecture. What is not subject to speculation is that both are epidemic for people already suffering from diabetes.

The uncertainty about autonomic neuropathy, its underlying causes, proper treatment and long-term prognosis sparked much of my desire to learn all I could about the disease and what it meant for me. I learned that Johnny Cash suffered from diabetes, developed autonomic neuropathy and died from the latter. I understood that in some situations, for some reasons, some of us progress from "manageable" autonomic neuropathy to pan autonomic failure and the shutdown of most vital systems. I listened well to the warnings from Dr, Syncope about the importance of maintain a positive attitude, being careful not to exacerbate the condition and to be religious about my sleep and medications - whatever combination of drugs that seemed to work at the time.

The first person who ever asked me why I fought all of this so hard and ended up with a personal breakthrough, and this book, was my editor. Margee caught me off guard with the question, not because the question is odd, but because, oddly, no one had ever asked me. I didn't have an answer. I am still pondering the great question.

Likely there are many reasons for the drive that pushed me to this point. Ask me to pick out one alone and I have to go with "pain."

I am a wimp. Always have been. I hate pain. Really hate pain. My life with unmanaged autonomic neuropathy came down to waking up to pain, with my only real goal for the day being how best I could manage the level of pain before going back to sleep.

As did my mother, I have believed in some form of near immortality since my youth, Well, as long as living to 100 counts as some form of immortality. My mother fell short by 20 years. Whether I make it past her milestone, let alone the Willard Scott Smuckers' moment, remains to be seen. Trust me, though, if my choice comes down to one of coming up short or living longer with the autonomic neuropathy pain I endured for years, I hope the check out time will come sooner rather than later.

In Detail

Vasoconstrictor — a drug that narrows the interior wall (lumen) of blood vessels. In the absence of a drug, your blood vessels narrow (constrict) or enlarge (dilate) constantly to increase/decrease blood flow along with increasing/decreasing blood pressure.

You experience vasoconstriction naturally when your body gets cold. In an effort to retain heat for internal organs, the vessels in your hands and feet — as well as those all along the skin's surface, will constrict to reduce blood flow. Getting hot? Your body goes through the opposite change: blood vessels dilate to increase the flow so that you release heat.

To understand the relationship between blood flow and pressure, consider the lowly garden hose. Turn on the water and grasp the end of the hose without a nozzle. Pinch the hose close to the opening and two things will happen. The amount of water (flow) will decrease and the pressure will increase.

One of the key mechanisms in your blood for controlling blood pressure, therefore, is the constriction and dilation of your vessels. As your blood vessels dilate, flow is increased as the pressure decreases. Constrict the vessels and flow decreases as the pressure increases. Of course, your heart plays an equally important role in these processes: an increased heart rate also assists in increasing blood flow. With a lower heart rate, just the opposite occurs.

Within the context of the book so far, this mechanism is important for two reasons: to understand better how a tilt-table test works and how vasoconstrictors reduce pain.

TILT-TABLE TEST

As warm-blooded animals, our body's ability to regulate core temperature is a wondrous asset that allows us to function in a variety of climates. Fish and reptiles, on the other hand, are cold-blooded and depend on environmental factors to maintain proper body temperature.

As an intelligent species, we rely on the same flow/pressure mechanism to keep our brains functioning under normal and extreme conditions. Under stress (be it physical, mental or emotional), our bodies do whatever possible to protect and preserve a sufficient flow of oxygen-enriched flow to the brain. Impair that flow to any significant extent and your brain begins to shut down. You start to feel lightheaded and, if the impairment increases, you'll faint.

During a tilt-table test, as the table pivots with your body into an upright position, your body works hard to keep the blood flowing at a proper rate to your head and brain. It does so by moving blood from your lower part of your body, particularly the legs. The vessels in your legs constrict helping to force more blood to other areas of your body.

However, if you suffer from a faulty flow/pressure mechanism, the vessels in your legs may not constrict enough and there is not sufficient blood flow to your brain. Rapidly falling heart rates or, as in my case, the cessation of a heartbeat, further impairs the flow of critical oxygenated blood to the brain.

NEUROPATHY

The faulty flow/pressure mechanism furthers complicates the daily lives of many patients with autonomic neuropathy. For reasons not well understood, our bodies work overtime to lower blood pressure through vessel dilation. This persistent dilation results in swelling and pain in the tissue surrounding blood vessels. It hurts. For many, it means a life of 24/7 pain from head to toe.

Vasoconstrictors offer one important way to manage episodes of severe pain. The key drawback is that too frequent use can cause a "rebound effect" where the vessels swell even further and/or the constriction cycle is reduce in time. As with many other sufferers, I used drugs that have strong vasoconstriction effects, such as Imitrex[1] and Frova[2], when the pain in my head merited more attention than other parts of the body. Both medications are generally prescribed for migraine headache attacks.

I found Frova to be very effective with fewer side effects than Imitrex. However, for more severe headaches, Imitrex seemed to work faster and better. For very rapid onset of an episode of severe pain, an injection of Imitrex, as opposed to a tablet, worked best for me.

Neurontin. One of the mostly commonly prescribed medications, Neurontin[3] provides autonomic neuropathy patients with sustained relief prior to and during episodes of nerve pain. Neurontin is approved by the FDA for treating pain related to shingles. Many autonomic neuropathy patients rely on this medication, but often need increasingly larger doses to manage the pain.

I found Neurontin to be an effective treatment in taking the edge off the pain and reducing the general discomfort to a manageable level. It never prevented or eliminated pain completely. And, Neurontin does have an unpleasant side effect: diminished mental function. I felt a bit "drugged out" with Neurontin. Not a terrible feeling, but I found it to slow my ability to think. So, it is a trade off. Less pain is good; less mental focus isn't.

TREATING AND LIVING WITH NEUROPATHY

Peripheral. Though there are many forms of peripheral neuropathy the greatest number of cases deal are associated with diabetes. Treating this form of neuropathy focuses on maintaining target glucose levels, avoiding cuts and sore on the feet as well managing the pain with a variety of medications. Neurontin is commonly used in pain treatment as well as some antidepressants and anticonvulsants. All are of limited effectiveness over time.

If you have peripheral neuropathy you should be careful not to injure your feet and feet – especially at the onset of numbness. Without a sense of pain, prolonged rubbing and scraping could lead to blisters and sores that do not heal. In prolonged cases, amputation of the affected limb could result.

Autonomic. The rule in dealing effectively with autonomic neuropathy is to find and work carefully with a doctor or medical team that understands your condition and with which you are comfortable. Effectively treating and living successfully with the disease involves long-term patience and care. Depending on the type and severity of the neuropathy, your treatment can involve several areas of focus:

Non-Drug and Lifestyle Treatments

- **Sleeping on an angle with your head raised.** This seems to help tolerate standing up in the morning. I also found in helpful in reducing snoring.

- **Increase salt intake.** Love chips and salsa? Eat up. OK, you still should watch the carbs and fat, but go for the salt. High salt intake tends to increase blood volume and helps in maintaining sufficient pressure. Sometimes drugs are prescribed to help in retaining salt.

- **Eat smaller meals.** Eating less at one sitting and going for frequent smaller meals shows up as a recommended treatment for the disorders covered in this book. In the case of autonomic neuropathy, a large meal leads to shunting the blood to the digestive system and away from other parts of the body. This can worsen the problems in balancing blood pressure throughout your body.

■ **Compression socks/hose.** The pressure of elastic socks and stockings on your lower legs tends to decrease blood pooling and can help some patients maintain a more balanced blood pressure.

■ **More caffeine.** Drinking coffee, tea and cola that all contain caffeine can help maintain blood pressure due to the vasoconstricting impact of caffeine. Some patients, however, find the added anxiety and jitters that can result are not worth the relief.

■ **Watch temperature extremes.** Many patients cannot tolerate hot days and rooms due to inability to sweat properly. Others cannot tolerate cold due to inadequate constricting of blood vessels. I fell into the former situation and it is scary. We sweat when the temperature goes up. We sweat to give off heat and our body cools. When you don't sweat and can't sense temperatures properly, you have the sense that all is well until the symptoms of heat exhaustion set in without warning. It becomes hard to mentally focus and you just can't think. Without help getting to cooler temperatures, you're going to be in serious trouble. The best advice: avoid temperature extremes.

- **Try exercising.** Some patients benefit from the physiological results of exercise. Others don't. If you are having problems sweating and/or keeping the blood pressure balanced from head to toe, try swimming. Being flat on your stomach or back in the water lessens stress on the blood pressure balancing mechanisms while the added pressure of the water keeps blood from pooling. In addition, the water surrounding your skin helps to keep your body cooler.

- **Drink water.** For many, additional water helps to maintain blood volume and pressure.

- **Know your limits.** You can't do everything you want. Accept that with grace, but don't give in and do nothing. Keep pushing the limits sensibly.

Drug Treatments

- Among the many types of medications that are used in managing autonomic neuropa-thy:

    - Salt-retaining steroids

- Beta-blockers (commonly used in treating cardiovascular disorders)

- Selective Serotonin Reuptake Inhibitors (SSRIs, commonly used as antidepressants)

- Clonodine, Midrodine and other vaso-constrictors

- Imitrex, Frova and other treatments for migraine headaches

MY APPROACH TO AUTONOMIC NEUROPATHY

My best advice as difficult as it may be: deal with the pain first and get it under control. Then, tackle one complication at a time with one medication. Find what works best for you without making a previously managed problem worse. It takes a long time to master your treatment if you suffer from multiple autonomic neuropathy complications.

In Addition

To learn more about treatments for neuropathy:

■ Search

- "Treatments for Diabetic Neuropathy," <u>Wrong Diagnosis,</u> November 15, 2006, < http://www.wrongdiagnosis.com/d/diabetic_neuropathy/treatments.htm>.

- "Antioxidant Soothes Diabetic Neuropathy," <u>WedMD</u>, 2006, < http://www.webmd.com/content/article/63/72066.htm>.

- "Neuropathy," <u>Health Communities.com</u>, September 2006, < http://www.answers.com/main/ntquery?s=neuropathy+treatme nts&gwp=13>.

▓ Endnotes

1. "Imitrex," <u>Migraine Relief Center</u>, GlaxoSmithKline, 2006 < http://www.migrainehelp.com/>.

2. "Frova," Endo Pharmaceuticals 2006 < http://www.frova. com/>.

3. "Neurontin," Pfizer 2006 < http://www.neurontin.com/>.

You can locate updated information
and additional links by visiting:
www.type4diabetes.com.

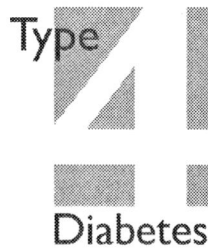

Type **4**
Diabetes

Chapter 4

- Cholesterol & Glucose

- Heart Disease & Diabetes

Chapter 4
Warnings About Cholesterol and Glucose

Dr. Syncope has few peers in the optimism department. I don't know of any doctors, let alone patients, who consistently muster the same warm smile and encouragement in spite of their own problems. His attitude is amazing and so welcome. I actually looked forward to each visit, despite the length of travel time to get to the center.

I won't forget a very cautious tone setting in, one day even with his gentle smile, as he strongly encouraged me to "keep my health up" and to do whatever possible I could to avoid two diseases: coronary heart disease and diabetes. "Get either of those," he warned, "and your life is going to become unbelievably more complicated." As if it wasn't already. I got the message.

So on a cold winter day in 2005, I started shivering from more than the weather as Dr. Internal cautioned me about my still rising cholesterol numbers. "Not something you want to deal with," he noted, in a nod to my other doctor's advice. "We need to do something."

Great. Let's add more medications to the daily menu. Some meals already seem to consist of a large plate of pills and a smaller one of food. Yummy.

Cholesterol. It comes from both your "Uncle Fat" and your "Fast Food."

OK. We attacked the "Fast Food" side of the equation

first through a drug called Zetia as well as changing my diet. Not that my diet qualified as American Awful, but for those whose cholesterol problem can be controlled through diet it is the place to start.

Good news for the "comfort food craver" in me: my bad cholesterol is not the result of diet. On the other hand, that's bad news for my desire not to add more drugs to my routine.

My cholesterol battle, though, merits no further attention except that it set into motion a chain of events that lead to my breakthrough in neuropathy management. Had it not been for the cholesterol issue there would have been no reason for repeated blood tests in 2005. And, without all those no-breakfast blood tests, it would have been a long time before I knew that I also had a problem with the glucose level in my blood.

So on a warm summer day in mid 2005, Dr. Internal patted me on the back for improving my cholesterol numbers (temporarily as it turned out) and then gently dropped a verbal bomb, "But we did find a different problem in your test. And it might be serious."

The problem: my fasting (prebreakfast) glucose reading indicated "prediabetes" — generally defined as being over 100 mg/dl. (For those unfamiliar with glucose measuring, please refer to 'In Detail" section later in this chapter.)

My doctor admitted surprise at seeing this test and cautioned that another test would be needed to confirm. One bright note, he added, was that a high glucose level could help to explain an odd occurrence of thrush (a fungal infection, not the bird) that occurred in my mouth five months previous. My having never experienced thrush before and with no other observable reason or test result to explain its appearance, Dr. Internal had no answers for me about the source of the fungus. Perhaps, he said, the thrush was an early warning signal about diabetes.

Thrush, though, generally appears after years of diabetes, not with someone getting a first test result of prediabetes or a diagnosis of Type 2 diabetes. And, Dr. Internal noted, he had not noticed any other indicators over the previous years that would lead him to conclude that I had a glucose problem or that I would likely be diagnosed with diabetes at my age. He knew that I exercised in spite of the autonomic neuropathy, kept my weight under control and had no apparent family history of diabetes.

Well, not so fast on the family part, though I didn't say anything at the time. He completed the exam and admonished me to "not wig out." Which is exactly what I did — even if I could not have told you what the word meant at the time. Deliriously excited, completely wild.

Don't get coronary artery disease. Don't get diabetes. I freaked. Fortunately.

My doctor may have forgotten, but I didn't. My mother had Type 2 diabetes. My doctor didn't know, but I did: my brother died from coronary complications due to diabetes less than 12 months previously.

I stumbled around the rest of the day and a few after that, to be honest. Living with the 24/7 pain and everything else associated with neuropathy presented enough misery, thank you. Now this! Not fair, damn it. I didn't wait for the subsequent tests to confirm Type 2. I knew what the tests would indicate, be it the next week or the next month or later.

Specialists in dealing with serious diseases frequently cite some variation on the five-stage Kübler-Ross Grief Cycle: denial, anger, bargaining, depression and acceptance. In no way I am demeaning the importance or relevance of this concept in saying that I blew through the first four stages and landed quickly in the fifth, acceptance, but with an interesting twist.

My ever-supportive family played an important role in this process. "Deal with it," was the general response. You're coping with other problems. Just do the same with this. Oh, so much easier said than done. But, the tough-love approach proved crucial in supporting my take charge attitude.

OK, I am going to deal with this, but in my own way. I am going to be obsessive about every aspect of this. I am going to learn everything possible about diabetes and do everything I can to beat it back. I focused on the future, but with a nagging interest in the past. Why now? Why were there no indications earlier? Does this have anything to do with autonomic neuropathy?

On the latter point, I suddenly recalled something my friend with neuropathy had asked me about nine months earlier. Do you have diabetes, yet?

What had he meant by 'yet' and why had he asked me the question? Why? His doctors (at another research center) had concluded that "nearly all" patients with autonomic neuropathy come down with diabetes within five years or so after diagnosis. So ...

In the weeks and months ahead I raided the local and online bookstores, bought any relevant magazines and Googled late into the night. As luck would have it, one of my first acquisitions in this area was an outstanding book by Dr. Anne Peters, director of the University of Southern California clinical diabetes programs. Her 2005 book, *Conquering Diabetes: A Cutting-Edge Comprehensive Program for Prevention and Treatment,*[1] merits must-read status for anyone facing diabetes either as a patient or care-giver.

Dr. Peters offers amazingly useful insights wrapped in an approach that spoke directly to my state of mind then and now: conquer diabetes. While serving up a bounty of easily understood answers to obvious questions, she spells out numerous questions that still remain to be addressed and casts some doubt on a few previously accepted "facts".

Not only does she present complex information clearly, she weaves in relevant stories from her patients, both famous and not. Among the former is Gary Hall, Jr., an Olympic gold medal winner for the US who discovered in 1999 that he had Type 1 while training for the 2000 Sydney games. Told by his doctors that he would never compete again, he sought out his own path, secured the assistance of Dr. Peters in managing diabetes and went on to win gold in Sydney. In 2004, he became the oldest US male (at 29) in 80 years to win a gold medal as he defended his 50m freestyle swimming title. His determination not to let diabetes, testing and insulin thwart his ambitions is truly inspirational.

I am neither an Olympic swimmer nor someone dealing with Type 1 and insulin. I am just an avid swimmer and I have to deal with Type 2 plus autonomic neuropathy. We each have lessons to share and help others.

Buoyed to a great extent by her book, I renewed my quest in earnest to solve as many mysteries as I could about my own situation. How to deal with it most effectively on a daily basis and what steps would be necessary in the longer term to afford me the quality of life I desired.

In Detail

Glucose and cholesterol. Diabetes and cardiovascular disease. Regardless of whether you label the problems by the more benign substance names or use the more frightening disease terminology, they are scary topics for an aging population.

Unfortunately, most of us treat them as two separate problems. In reality, they intertwine, presenting a messy challenge to sustained good health in middle age and beyond. If you get one, you're likely to incur the other. That's sad since two out of three people with diabetes die from heart disease and stroke.[2] In addition, people with diabetes are:

- 2-4 time more likely to have a heart attack or stroke as someone without diabetes[3]

- Nearly all people with diabetes have abnormally high cholesterol levels.[4]

- People with diabetes have the same risk of dying from a heart attack as someone who already has had a heart attack

Why? The answers are both easy, on a basic level, and very complex in terms of long-term effective treatment. At the risk of being overly simplistic, high blood glucose levels seem to exacerbate the potential for cholesterol-produced plaque to form on artery walls. On the other side, the reduction in physical activity, common with cardiovascular patients, is considered to a major factor in the onset of Type 2 diabetes. The detailed mechanisms involved are likely to be far more complex.

In spite of all these statistics, nearly 70% of patients with diabetes aren't aware of the increased risk for stroke and heart disease. [5]

Thankfully, both the American Heart Association[6] and the American Diabetes Association[7] spend considerable time and money on changing perceptions of the diabetes and coronary heart disease.

"Diabetes dramatically increases a person's risk for heart disease and stroke and often is associated with other cardiovascular risk factors, such as high blood pressure, cholesterol disorders, obesity and insulin resistance. Unfortunately, most people with diabetes are not aware of these prevalent health risks."[8]

"Most people with diabetes have health problems -- or risk factors -- such as high blood pressure and cholesterol that increase one's risk for heart disease and stroke. When combined with diabetes, these risk factors add up to big trouble. In fact, more than 65% of people with diabetes die from heart disease or stroke. With diabetes, heart attacks occur earlier in life and often result in death. By managing diabetes, high blood pressure and cholesterol, people with diabetes can reduce their risk

Nearly all people with diabetes have abnormal cholesterol levels which contribute to their increased risk for heart attack and stroke. By choosing foods wisely, increasing physical activity and taking medications, you can improve your cholesterol."[9]

Both groups offer comprehensive education programs to help Americans understand just how critical it is to focus on both diabetes and heart disease, regardless of your present health. The Heart Association offers an entire site, The Heart of Diabetes, full of information on steps that can be taken to lower the risks of both diabetes and cardiovascular disease. Included on this site is a program where you can track your glucose, blood pressure and cholesterol. It's worth spending time viewing. [10]

Did you know ... The Heart Of Diabetes Family History Tree: Like the color of your eyes, tendencies for many health condi-

tions are genetically passed from one family member to another. The more you know about your family's health history, the more you can do to reduce your risk of diabetes and heart disease.[11]

Similarly, the American Diabetes Association offers a special site: "Make the Link! Diabetes, Heart Disease and Stroke."[12]

Make the Link! stresses that diabetes management is more than control of blood glucose. People with diabetes must also manage blood pressure and cholesterol and talk to their health care provider to learn about other ways to reduce their chance for heart attacks and stroke.

Among the numerous health features on the site is an interactive section called: For People with Diabetes and their Loved Ones."

In this section, you will learn how you can prevent heart attacks and stroke. Read the new Diabetes Survival Guide, a resource to help you make good choices and learn what you need to know to take care of your diabetes. You can also view Link for Life starring Type 2 Lou, a fun, interactive program filled with practical tips and valuable information. Link for Life is available in both English & Spanish.

PREVENTION AND TREATMENT

The National Institutes of Health (NIH) is engaged in several studies aimed at lowering the rate of cardiovascular disease in people with diabetes. Among those studies[13]:

1. Action for Health in Diabetes (Look AHEAD) focuses on voluntary weight loss

2. Action to Control Cardiovascular Risk in Diabetes (ACCORD) is studying three different approaches:

    a. More intensive glucose control

    b. More intensive blood pressure control

    c. Use of medication to lower triglyceride levels while raising HDL (good) cholesterol

These studies along with dozens more at other research centers, will take place for years before statistically valid results can be obtained. Until then, the best road to take seems to be three-pronged:

1. Loss weight

2. Increase exercise

3. Stay informed

In Addition

To learn more about the link between glucose and cholesterol, diabetes and cardiovascular disease:

▮ Read

- Diabetes and Heart Healthy Cookbook, (Arlington, VA: American Diabetes Association, 2003)

▮ Search

- "Make the Link: Diabetes, Heart Disease and Stroke," Diabetes, < http://www.diabetes.org/heart-disease-stroke.jsp>.

- "Diabetes, Heart Disease, and Stroke," National Diabetes Information Clearinghouse, December 2005, < http://diabetes. niddk.nih.gov/dm/pubs/stroke/#connection>.

- "The Heart of Diabetes," American Heart Association, 2005, < http://www.s2mw.com/heartofdiabetes/>.

- "Diabetes and cardiovascular disease: Lifestyle changes and medication can improve your health," CNN, May 2005, < http://www.cnn.com/HEALTH/library/DA/00052.html>.

◼ Endnotes

1. Anne Peters, Conquering Diabetes (New York: Hudson Street Press, 2005)

2. "Make The Link! Diabetes, Heart Disease and Stroke," American Diabetes Association, 2006 < http://diabetes.org/heart-disease-stroke.jsp>.

3. "Diabetes and cardiovascular disease: Lifestyle changes and medication can improve your health," CNN Health/Library 2006 < http://www.cnn.com/HEALTH/library/DA/00052. html>.

4. "Make The Link!"

5. "Diabetes and cardiovascular disease:"

6. American Heart Association <http://www.geart.org>.

7. American Diabetes Associaton <http://www.diabetes.org>.

8. "Heart of Diabetes," American Heart Association 2006 < http://www.s2mw.com/heartofdiabetes/index.html>.

9. "Make The Link!"

10. "Heart Healthy Tracker," <u>American Heart Association</u> 2006 < http://www.s2mw.com/AHA/usercentral.aspx>.

11. "Heart Healthy Tracker"

12. "Make The Link!"

13. "Diabetes Overview," <u>National Diabetes Information Clearing-</u><u>house (NDIC)</u> 2006 < http://diabetes.niddk.nih.gov/dm/pubs/ overview/index.htm>.

You can locate updated information
and additional links by visiting:
www.type4diabetes.com.

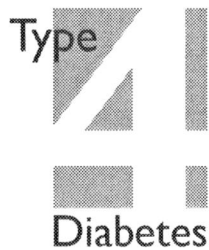

Chapter 5

- Prediabetes

- Type 1 Diabetes

- Type 2 Diabetes

Chapter 5
Diagnosis of Diabetes

Growing up in 50s and 60s, I recall hushed, solemn conversations between my parents when a neighbor or friend was discovered to be "spilling" water or sugar. My mother would wring her hands, shake her head and intone "tragic, just tragic."

Given their careers, cocktail-hour discussions invariably led to some comments about a disease or medical procedure, usually in coded vernacular popular at the time. A diagnosis of cancer was termed as "having the C." Mental illness merited a "not right" euphemism. Abortion, "that *very private* procedure." Develop diabetes and you were spilling something.

I never got around to asking my parents before they passed why all the coded language. Were they trying to protect the three kids from sad realities of mortal bodies? Or did they, even as medical professionals, find some things too scary? I suspect a combination of both lay at the root of the language conventions.

Given the state of medicine at the time in dealing with life-threatening chronic diseases, fear was understandable.

Prior to 1922 and the first use of insulin in humans, a childhood diagnosis of Type 2 diabetes equated to a death sentence. An incredibly strict diet could prolong life expectancy, but not for long nor with a reasonable quality of life. Patients came close to starving under the diet and some form of organ failure set in sooner or later.

Insulin was the first dramatic step in managing diabetes and, for those who could afford it, a true life-saver. The cost of insulin use, however, was not measured only in dollars, but also in determining the right dosage at the right time. Too little over time and the ravages of diabetes, though delayed, would set in: blindness, kidney failure, amputations due to sores not healing. A missed dose or an ineffective dose —the wrong combination of food intake and energy output — could result in ketoacidosis and lead to sudden death

On the other side of the equation, injecting too much insulin presented doctors at the time with a new problem: hypoglycemia, or low blood sugar. As the level of glucose drops below normal, the body begins to starve for fuel. Go too low and brain function will be impaired, with unconsciousness following. If the condition is not treated at this point, death can occur.

Imagine the plight of the patient and the doctors in the first 60 years after insulin introduction. We have this life-saving hormone, but we can't really tell you when its best to use it and how much to inject when you do. But, when you do use it, don't give yourself too much or too little.

What we accept as matter of fact, handheld glucose meters, simple didn't exist. Prior to the advent of meters in 1980, a urine test was the only reliable method for ascertaining too high a level of glucose. Lab-based urine analysis was just a more measured diagnostic approach to the same test used by the ancient Greeks and Romans. Physicians at the time tasted a patient's urine. If it tasted sweet, the patient had diabetes, a word coined in the 1st century CE.

Thankfully, for both health and aesthetic reasons, we are past that era now.

Realize, though, that even the best urine tests could not determine if someone's glucose level was too low. So, it's only been in the last 25 years that adequate tools have been available for tracking and understanding the downside of the diabetes curve: hypoglycemia. There is a lot we simply don't know — yet.

Meters and test strips rightfully occupy a permanent place in the lives of anyone with diabetes, or even prediabetes. We all react differently to the same food, the same exercise, the same stress. If we are to achieve the control necessary for managing diabetes, let alone conquering it, we must understand our own glucose levels as they rise and fall.

Armed with my newly acquired LifeScan OneTouch Ultra meter and a packet of $1 per test strips, I set out on the same path millions undertake each year. I began with the fasting (pre-breakfast) test and then progressed to testing after breakfast and at different times of the day. I'll admit to a sense of fascination in watching how my glucose level rose and fell at different times of the day.

Chow down on some pancakes and syrup for breakfast and watch it soar. Be good, cut back on the carbs and relax as it settles down. It doesn't take long to note basic trends. It is comforting to realize that the generally accepted guidance for food intake works for you as well.

What is more interesting, though, is getting an increasingly detailed insight into why you have "unexplained" highs. Unexplained meaning that you haven't determined the lag time yet for your body's response to elevated energy need (exercise) and decreased carbohydrate consumption.

It is at this junction that I discovered a variance of opinion among doctors concerning home testing for prediabetes and, in some cases, even for Type 2 diabetes. For a bevy of reasons, some doctors advise against home testing for people with prediabetes or recently diagnosed Type 2. Oft heard or read are expressions of concern that patients will become fixated on the home tests and the rapid glucose level changes and miss the important considerations of focusing on diet and exercise. Some doctors seem to avoid the issue of home testing out of consideration that many Type 2 patients are burdened enough with just dealing with the emotional aspects of having a chronic disease. Testing just might "overload" some patients to the point of "shutting down" about the whole topic.

Perhaps. I am more inclined to accept concern for patients with a phobia to needles as being a more logical reason to shy away from daily testing. Even then, I can't accept any reason for not encouraging every person who even is suspected of becoming diabetic to engage in regular home testing. My opinion.

If a needle drives you mad, then have someone else test your blood somewhere else other than your sensitive fingertips Be sure to select testing and lancing devices that minimize the discomfort. Look away while the test is being done. Get a therapist to work with you on coping with the phobia. Better to do this now and control the diabetes than do nothing and end up relying on insulin injections that are more painful than a "stick in the arm."

Luckily, I don't have any fear of needles or my own blood. Whatever discomfort and reluctance I might have had about pricking myself quickly disappeared early in my battle with autonomic neuropathy. At the time it was either inject myself or endure a level 8+ headache for 1-2 days. Pain, indeed, can modify one's behavior quickly.

I do have an elevated curiosity about most things. My mother used to admonish me regularly for "being jack of all trades and master of none." To which I rejoined, "I prefer to call myself a Renaissance Man, thank you."

I am also a geek, a nerd. Tried and true. Down to the very core of my being.

So, there I sat one evening early in my days with the glucose meter, intrigued by how it worked — and annoyed that it had to be manually coded for different strips. Please. How hard could that be to pull off?

Moving past the somewhat trivial, a familiar itch developed, the same one that generally occurs whenever I pick up something that could be called a gadget. Anything with a battery and some silicon qualifies. My family even has a name for all these items and my affection for them, "Bob-O-Matic." I love my toys. But, I don't want them to just do basic things, I want to get everything I can out of a Bob-O-Matic toy.

In the case of the LifeScan meter, I noticed a port on one side (a small outlet for the normal people reading this section). The port meant a connection to a larger computer. A larger computer meant I could grab all the data from these tests and play with them (model then in my lingo). Oh, boy. Charts and graphs, here we come. To what end, one might ask? As if something concrete or meaningful was actually that important to me. Why did I want to play with data? Because I could.

In Detail

As noted in the introduction to this book, if you are reading this book you know that diabetes is a serious disease involving faulty glucose metabolism. More than most, you also know that diabetes, if not treated properly, is also a leading cause of adult blindness, amputations and kidney failure. And, it significantly increases your chance for cardiovascular disease. Diabetes is scary and dangerous.

It is also manageable. Thankfully. Learning that you have diabetes, or prediabetes, is no longer a death sentence as it was in the days before insulin. Diabetes no longer means a shortened life expectancy or even daily misery — if you are diagnosed early and take care of yourself.

This may come as a shock, but diabetes is also an exciting disease. Incredible strides have been made in the understanding and treatment of this disease. More than any other disease, research has proven that most people can control the disease through lifestyle changes and without the need for medications. We can only hope that one day most diseases could be managed by making adjustments to our diets and level of physical activity.

Everyone who is now diagnosed with diabetes owes a great deal of thanks to the thousands of women and men in the medical field, the drug industry, at research centers and in educational groups such as the American Diabetes Association. They have made our lives so much easier and promise an even brighter future.

Given all of that, though, it is nearly incomprehensible to learn that:

■ About 21 million people in the US have diabetes (about 7% of the population)[1]

■ Each year, more than 1.5 million people aged 20 and older are diagnosed with diabetes

■ More than 90% of those diagnosed each year have Type 2, the "controllable" and perhaps "preventable" form

■ And yet, more than 6.2 million people do not know they have this serious, lifelong condition.

If you have diabetes, think you may have diabetes or are a care-giver for someone who does, there are many outstanding books, websites and other reference materials you should consider reading and viewing. I offer just a sample of them at the end of this chapter. Let me, though, provide you with a solid overview.

WHAT IS DIABETES?

According to the National Institute of Diabetes and Digestive and Kidney Diseases (NIDDK), a part of the National Institutes of Health:

Diabetes is a disorder of metabolism
– the way our bodies use digested food for growth and energy.

Most of the food we east is broken down into glucose, the form of sugar in the blood. Glucose is the main source of fuel for the body.

After digestion, glucose passes into the bloodstream, where it is used by cells for growth and energy. For glucose to get into cells, insulin must be present. Insulin is a hormone produced by the pancreas, a large gland behind the stomach.

When we eat, the pancreas automatically produces the right amount of insulin to move glucose from blood into our cells. In people with diabetes, however, the pancreas either produces too little or no insulin, or the cells do not respond appropriately to the insulin that is produced. Glucose builds up in the blood, overflows into the urine and passes out of the body in the urine. Thus, the body loses its main source of fuel even though the blood contains large amounts of glucose.[2]

For the purposes of full disclosure, let me add that despite the stamp of approval from the US government, this definition of diabetes does not meet with complete unanimity within the worldwide medical community. Many distill the definition down to "a chronic condition with too much glucose in the blood." While I am in no position to contradict that shorter meaning, I do fault the implication that the focus of understanding about diabetes should just be on elevated levels of glucose.

The mechanisms involved in glucose metabolism and maintenance are exceedingly complex and still not well understood. The point of this book is to argue that the focus of diabetes research and treatment must expand beyond the "hills" of glucose to include the "valleys" as well.

THE TYPES OF DIABETES

Here again, there are agreements and disputes about classification.

Three types of diabetes are generally accepted:

- Type 1

- Type 2

- Gestational Diabetes

Type 1: an autoimmune disease where the body's system for fighting infection (the immune system) goes awry, attacks and destroys the insulin-producing beta cells in the pancreas. A person with Type 1 produces little or no insulin and, therefore, must take insulin daily to live. In most cases, a person with Type 1 injects herself with insulin one or more times each day. Increasingly, though, people with Type 1 diabetes prefer to manage their insulin levels with a pump worn around the waist. The FDA has recently approved the first inhaled insulin. Though it has it drawbacks, this landmark approach paves the way for additional therapies that do not involve the daily use of needles or or an external pump.

Type 2: In the past, this form of diabetes was referred to as "Adult Onset" or "Non-Insulin Dependent Diabetes." Both terms, unfortunately, are not correct. Increasingly, children are being diagnosed with Type 2 – most of the underlying cause due to improper diet and obesity. While people with Type 2 are most frequently treated with oral medications or lifestyle changes, as opposed to insulin, an ever increasing number must eventually turn to insulin to properly manage the disease.

In Type 2, the pancreas usually produces enough insulin, but for unknown reasons the body cannot use the insulin effectively. Something changes either in the insulin produced or in the way cells take in insulin from the blood. This change is labeled as "insulin resistance." The body works hard to overcome this change by producing greater amounts of insulin. After several years, the pancreatic cells producing insulin become "exhausted" by this over production and insulin production decreases. When this happens, glucose beings to build up in the blood – just as with Type 1.

Gestational Diabetes: Approximately 3-8% of women in the United States develop a form of diabetes late in pregnancies. After birth, most of these women have normal glucose levels again. However, recent studies have shown that 20-50% of women who have had this type of diabetes will develop Type 2 within 5 to 10 years.

You may also read about:

Type 1.5: It is argued by some researchers that at least 10% (perhaps as many as 20%) of people with Type 2 actually have a form of autoimmune-related diabetes.[3] Referred to as either Type 1.5 or Latent Autoimmune Diabetes in Adults (LADA), this type is often not diagnosed. When a child develops diabetes, it is assumed to be Type 1; with adults Type 2. In adults, regardless of whether it is Type 2 or Type 1.5, the treatment progression is generally the same: lifestyle changes, oral medications and then insulin.

Type 1.5 patients do not have insulin resistance so certain medications will prove ineffective and your doctor will try to prescribe something else. That is the essence of the controversy of whether to formally recognize this type of diabetes with its own classification.

There are blood tests to make a diagnosis of Type 1.5 possible. In addition, Type 1.5 patients tend not to be overweight, are often physically fit, have low-normal tricglyceride levels, normal to high levels of HDL (good cholesterol) and normal blood pressure. Given these indicators, you can understand why this group of diabetes patients does not have the same risk factor as Type 2 for developing cardiovascular disease.

One important advantage of adding this classification to standard usage is the increased probability of getting the right medications sooner.

Type 3: discussed in detail in Chapter 6, "A New Name for Alzheimer's?", the Type 3 classification is being promoted by researchers at the Brown Medical School.

Type 4: a major focus of this book, the argument for Type 4 is presented in detail in Chapter 11. Type 4 is the conjunction of diabetes, autonomic neuropathy and hypoglycemia.

HOW IS DIABETES DIAGNOSED?

For Type 1 and Type 2 diabetes, the standards are:

TABLE 5-1 Glucose Levels for Determining Diabetes			
	US Plasma(1)	US Whole Blood(2)	International Plasma(3)	Internat. Whole Blood(4)
Before breakfast (after 8-hour fast)	126 or above	112 or above	7.0 or above	6.2 or above
Random test any time of day	200 or more	179 or above	11.1 or above	9.9 or above
(1) In the US, blood glucose is measured in milligrams per deciliter of plasma (a blood component) or whole blood. Laboratory testing provides results in plasma and these results are the standards for diagnosing diabetes.				
(2) Home meters test in whole blood. However, some meters display in "plasma equivalent." Be sure to check your meter, the instructions guide or contact the manufacturer to be sure how the meter is set or calibrated. Whole blood results are approximately 12% lower than plasma blood tests. Note that home testing meters are considered clinically accurate if it falls within +/20% of an accepted reference laboratory test. See Chapter 7 for more information.				
(3) In Canada, Europe and most other places outside of the US, glucose is typically measured in millimoles per liter.				
(4) If your International meter displays in whole blood, this is the approximate equivalent reading to standard plasma laboratory results.				

Oral Glucose Tolerance Test (OGTT): once a popular method for diagnosing diabetes, the OGTT is in less favor now with many doctors preferring fasting blood tests. The OGTT involves drinking a large glass of very sweet cola or juice and then testing for glucose levels in two hours. Some doctors, though, still prefer the test and it is often used for testing gestational diabetes and for determining subtle glucose metabolism problems.

WHAT IS PREDIABETES?

A diagnosis of prediabetes qualifies you as a member of one of the largest and fastest-growing "health concern clubs" in our society. According to the NIH, more than 54 million US adults had prediabetes in 2002.[1] It is more common in the US than in other countries due to our unhealthy diets and couch-potato approach to exercise.

The bad news about prediabetes is that you are likely to develop full-blown Type 2 unless you do something about it. The good news is that you can do a lot to prevent or delay the onset of diabetes.

Large-scale studies in the US and the UK, beginning in the 1990s, have clearly demonstrated that people a high risk for developing Type 2 can sharply lower that risk through diet and exercise. In fact, one study showed that a diet and exercise program resulted in a 5-7% weight loss and lowered the incidence of Type 2 by nearly 60%[2].

If your test results qualify you as having prediabetes, there are four major steps you should take:

1. Consult your doctor, if you have not already done so.

2. Learn as much as you can about prediabetes, what it means for you and what you can do to delay or prevent Type 2.

3. Begin a diet and exercise program.

4. Track your numbers with a home meter.

TABLE 5-2 Glucose Levels for Determining Prediabetes				
	US Plasma(1)	US Whole Blood(2)	International Plasma(3)	International Whole Blood(4)
Before breakfast (after 8-hour fast)	100-125	112 or above	5.5-6.9	4.9-6.1
(1) - (4) Please refer to Table 5-1				

In Addition

■ Read

- Anne Peters, <u>Conquering Diabetes</u> (New York, NY:Hudson Street Press, 2005)

- Paula Ford-Martin and Ian Blummer, <u>The Everything Diabetes Book</u> (Avon, MA: Adams Media, 2004)

- Alan L. Rubin, <u>Diabetes for Dummies</u> (Hoboken, NJ: Wiley, 2004)

- Julia Van Tine, ed., <u>Prevention: Outsmart Diabetes</u> (Rodale 2005)

- Gretchen Becker, <u>Type 2 Diabetes: An Essential Guide to the Newly Diagnosed</u> (New York: Marlowe & Company, 2001

■ **Search**

- "Diabetes," <u>CDC</u> < http://www.cdc.gov/diabetes/>.

- "Diabetes," <u>National Diabetes Information Clearing House</u> < http://diabetes.niddk.nih.gov/>.

- "Diabetes," <u>Medline</u> < http://www.nlm.nih.gov/medlineplus/diabetes.html>.

■ Visit (websites for periodicals and TV)

- <u>Diabetes Forecast</u>, American Diabetes Association < http://www.diabetes.org/diabetes-forecast.jsp>.

- <u>Diabetes Self-Management</u> < http://www.diabetesselfmanagement.com>.

- <u>Diabetes Health</u> < http://www.diabeteshealth.com/>.

- <u>Diabetic Living</u> < http://www.bhg.com/bhg/store/product.jhtml?catid=cat3860016&prodid=prd553180>.

- <u>dLife</u> (TV) < http://www.dlife.com/>.

■ Endnotes

1. "Diabetes Overview," <u>National Diabetes Information Clearinghouse</u>, 2006 < http://diabetes.niddk.nih.gov/dm/pubs/overview/index.htm>.

2. "Diabetes Overview"

3. JP Palmer, et al, "Is latent autoimmune diabetes in adults distinct from type 1 diabetes or just type 1 diabetes at an older age?" <u>NCBI PubMed</u>, December 2005, < Is latent autoimmune diabetes in adults distinct from type 1 diabetes or just type 1 diabetes at an older age?>

4. "Diabetes Overview"

5. "Diabetes Overview"

You can locate updated information
and additional links by visiting:
www.type4diabetes.com.

Type **4** Diabetes

Chapter 6

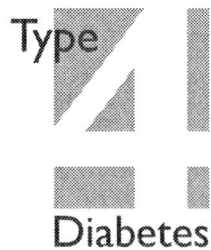

■ Alzheimer's Disease

Chapter 6
Type 3 Diabetes: A New Name for Alzheimer's?

At first glance, many will wonder why Alzheimer's Disease is even mentioned in a book on diabetes, let alone given an entire chapter inserted into the middle of the flow. Good question. A few months ago I surely would have expressed the same puzzlement.

Many remarkable events filled the months of 2006 as I researched the foundation concepts of Type 4 Diabetes. You will read about these in the coming chapters. If you are jumping directly to this chapter, I invite — encourage — you to read the book in its entirety even if your interest is focused on Alzheimer's.

As I conceived this book, the working title was "The Dangerous Downside of Diabetes." I appreciated the fact that the foundations of my research suggested a reexamination of the classification of diabetes into differing types, but didn't dwell on how the link could or should fit into the existing system focusing on Type 1 and Type 2.

Then my research led me to the remarkable work of Dr. Suzanne de la Monte and her colleagues at Brown Medical School — along with a growing cadre of experts around the world — linking Alzheimer's Disease with diabetes. The obvious potential for this work is truly staggering.

Based on this work, Dr. de la Monte has proposed renaming Alzheimer's "Type 3 Diabetes." Only time will tell if that label meets with long-term acceptance. Reading about the efforts to tame Alzheimer's with diabetes' treatments proved to be a seminal point in my writing. As you will read later in this chapter, the Brown research and discoveries mandate a new look on how diabetes is defined and its implications for tens of millions around the world. Before the "In Detail" section, I offer my personal, tragic experience with Alzheimer's and why that experience reinforces the foundation of this book.

The Journey Continues...

Often heard around the Alzheimer's care-giver community is the phrase "36-Hour Day." The term strongly conveys the incredible stress laid on family and friends in caring for people with Alzheimer's disease. If you have a loved one with this terrible disease you understand. If you are fortunate to not as yet have someone you love succumb, be prepared.

Your first clue that something is wrong with a friend or family member frequently occurs in an oddly humorous fashion. Something goofy happens that defies reasonable explanation. In the case of my mother, that first warning came during an overnight flight from Atlanta to Germany in 1985. Having served in World War II as an aide to Gen. Patton, my dad wanted to return to the places where he had been stationed. The paternal side of my mother's family came from Heidelberg and she had never been back to search for her heritage.

The trip had been long planned and eagerly anticipated. My college German proved to be a tad rusty, but adequate for the task of getting my father out of frequent trouble when he would loudly complain "Everyone should be speaking English. After all, we won that damn war!" That approach proved especially charming in über-nationalistic Bavaria.

It was my mother, though, who got the trip off to a flying start on the L1011 widebody. Proud of myself for planning so far ahead, I had reserved the two side seats right behind one of the mid-plane doors for my parents. All the legroom anyone would want and no seats flopping back in their faces. Good plan. Bad timing.

My mother spent the entire night trying to open the handle of the door in front of her so she could go outside for a smoke. I know that those door handles are set not to open during pressurized flight. Most people know that. What I couldn't be sure of was whether the handles "knew" that.

It was far from the first time my mother had flown in a jet and not even the first time over the Atlantic Ocean at night. My dad slept well, as usual. And I freaked out, also as usual.

I had never seen the far-away look in mother's face before. I couldn't get her to focus on her real location. Do you know where you are, Mom? She simply could not respond to the question. She just stared off into space as if trying to get her bearings that, I guess, she really was seeking.

When we left the plane in Frankfurt, my mother was less confused but unsettled. I resembled a sleep-deprived raccoon. My dad was well rested and looking forward to seeing America's Germany.

The trans-oceanic episode did not repeat itself on the trip back nor were there any significantly odd moments in my mother's behavior during the car trip through Germany, France, Switzerland and Austria.

I am glad for many reasons that we took the trip, as it turned out to be the last one for the three of us. The episode with my mother made me suspect something wrong. And upon return I paid careful attention to her actions and changes in personality. Within a few months, I expected the worst.

At the time, I lived in Atlanta and my parents resided south of Richmond, Virginia. Once I suspected the nature of her illness, I thought it would be little problem to convince my father to get my mother to her doctors. Wrong. Having quizzed my dad for weeks about my mother's behavior, he knew exactly where I thought the road would lead and he wanted none of it.

I'll take care of it, he assured me. It's not going to be a problem. I can handle it.

Courageous words for a man of 80. Brave words, though misplaced, for any man or women regardless of age. Caring for an Alzheimer's patient is beyond the capabilities of almost anyone. My dad learned that lesson the hard way very quickly as my mother's health deteriorated. Still, though, he was reluctant to seek the necessary advice and proper diagnosis from doctors.

It came down to moving my family back to Virginia so I could be close enough to juggle work and get my mother to her appointments. I should have been angrier at my dad, but I wasn't. Once again his medical background collided with his upbringing. He refused to take my mother to see any doctor. He wouldn't talk with her about the problem. And, when the diagnosis was confirmed, he extracted a promise from me not to tell any of the neighbors or relatives. My fingers were crossed.

I applied constant pressure to get him to consider one of the then new assisted living facilities — to no avail. He wouldn't even allow a nurse to visit the house once a week to check in. "I'll take care of it," he repeated unendingly. Aside from the myriad of problems that come with the emotional fireworks that accompany the progression of Alzheimer's, my dad was also ill equipped to handle even some basic chores. As kids, we joked that my dad had lost the recipe on how to boil water. He was handy everywhere else in the house, but the kitchen remained a total mystery to him.

Finally, the hunger from missing the same meals my mother insisted she had already consumed moved my father's stubbornness. Unfortunately, the real push came as a result of his own deteriorating health. He felt increasingly weak for reasons other than caring for my mother.

Not long after moving into the assisted living facility he was diagnosed with terminal lung cancer. And, at the time he gave the greatest gift a father could pass on to his son: the dignity that can be found in dying.

The final diagnosis curtailed a July 4th vacation. Flying back to Richmond, I spelled out the typical options of surgery and chemo. Unable to speak above a whisper at the time, he shook his head. "No. I have had a great life. It's time to go. Let all the family and friends know, help your mother understand and take care of her. Maybe I should have done something else for her when I could. I am sorry, son."

Nineteen days later he died peacefully. Called to the nursing home with hours left to go, I spent his last afternoon and evening by his side as he fell in and out of sleep. Each time he woke, we talked about our fun moments in incredible lucidity. He wanted only Tylenol for the pain. Being able to communicate with me until the end was vital to him. As the sun set, I asked him if he wanted to see my mother for the last time. He nodded yes and I went to the other part of the facility to wheel her down.

As we went into his room, I asked her if she knew why we were there. To say goodbye, she muttered. And they did.

During the night our conversation grew briefer and further apart. He woke up just before dawn, told me that he loved me and "thanks." And as the dawn's light came up, I witnessed his spirit depart.

Death with amazing dignity.

My mother had no such good fortune.

The evening of my father's passing was a complete 180° turn of events for me. Twenty-four hours earlier I sat peacefully with my father. Now, I sat by my mother's bedside listening all night long as she begged me to kill her. "If you really love me, Robert, you'll kill me right now. Please. Please. Please. You promised me as a kid never to let me end up in a mental asylum." True. The tears and the anguish for both of us are seared into my soul.

In all honesty, I timidly had brought the subject up with my dad just prior to moving into the facility. We both knew it could be done, essentially how to do it, and with his friends, where we could go for the medications. I knew we might one day regret not doing it, but even I couldn't bring myself to assist in her death. Given the terror she suffered through, I truly regret my inaction.

Trained in the 30's and 40's as a psychiatric nurse, my mother truly toiled in the Dark Ages of caring for mental illness - frontal lobotomies, ice baths, electro shocks. Too brutal even to contemplate. But for my mother, that was her past. And, as her memory unwound and disappeared last things first, she ended up really living in the past. She had no place to retreat in her mind. Just hell. And it was for her.

My mother died four years later with no options as to her own treatment and life/death choices, as my father had exercised. She died in a nursing home, bedridden, with no ability on my part to improve her environment or situation. At the time, health insurance generally disregarded Alzheimer's and refused to cover any treatment or care. Medicare was never enough and the whole experience, as it is for so many families, is a journey into financial chaos or ruin.

I have availed myself of this opportunity to discuss my mother, both out of respect as well as the stunning coincidence that occurred as I began work on this book. It came to my attention in the later years of my mother's life that she had also suffered from that "spilling water" disease. At the time I paid little attention to that fact. Her doctor told me it was finally under control, though the doctor did not know for how long my mother had been dealing with Type 2.

The onset and coping with her Alzheimer's made the diabetes a side issue. In light of all the new research, perhaps we all missed a critical component.

In July 2006, thousands of researchers gathered in Madrid for the Tenth International Conference on Alzheimer's Disease and Related Disorders. The headlines emerging from the conference focused on several reports and research projects, pointing a very incriminating finger at diabetes being a primary key to understanding Alzheimer's.

Among the reports: Swedish doctors wrote that people with high blood sugar levels were 70% more likely to develop Alzheimer's. An analysis of records at the US Veterans Affairs medical system suggested that certain Type 2 diabetes drugs may significantly lower the risk of Alzheimer's. A doctor at the University of Virginia noted some very early success in treating Alzheimer's patients with a specific Type 2 oral medication.

Researchers at Brown Medical School in Providence, Rhode Island, have taken to calling at least one form of Alzheimer's by a new name: Type 3 Diabetes.

In Detail

WHAT IS ALZHEIMER'S DISEASE?

Dementia is a brain disorder that seriously affects a person's ability to carry out daily activities. Alzheimer's disease is the most common form of dementia among older people — with an estimated four million Americans suffering from its cruelty. It involves the parts of the brain that control thought, memory, and language. Every day scientists learn more, but right now the causes of Alzheimer's disease are still unknown, and there is no cure.[1]

The disease bears the name of Dr. Alois Alzheimer, a German psychiatrist, who diagnosed the first recorded case in 1901. He showed his patient several objects and later asked her what she had been shown. She could not recall the objects — a test still used in some manner today to help in diagnosing the disease. When she died five years later, he worked with two Italian physicians to examine her brain structure. The discovery of the hallmark neurofibrillary tangles and amyloid plaques led to the classification of the disease as a specific form of dementia.

For most of the 20th Century, dementia was considered a natural part of aging and little attention was paid outside of neurological specialists to differentiating the forms of dementia. But, with the aging of the Western European and American populations, the focus began to shift in the 1970s and early 1980s to understanding the differences between dementia observed in elderly patients and those under 65. As this shift occurred, Dr. Alzheimer's disease achieved widespread recognition.

Alzheimer's disease begins slowly. Initially, symptoms

of mild forgetfulness are the only clues. Stress, disease, certain medications and aging all make us prone to forget things. Sometimes we forget why we went into a room. That is natural, though frustrating. Alzheimer's patients tend to forget that they even went into the room, let alone why.

As the disease progresses, these lapses become more frequent and more pronounced. People in later stages of the disease often forget how to simple tasks such as brushing their teeth, combing their hair or dialing a phone. They just cannot think clearly any more. They begin to have problems with language: speaking, understanding, writing and reading become difficult. Anxiousness, aggressiveness or wandering away from home may occur. At some point, total 24/7 care is required.

Life expectancy is usually 7-10 years for a patient from the date of diagnosis.

HOW IS IT DIAGNOSED?

The only definite way to completely determine Alzheimer's is the same as it was 100 years ago – perform an autopsy on the brain. However, neurologists use a variety of tests to arrive at a diagnosis of "possible" or "probable" Alzheimer's disease:

- Cognitive memory tests (similar to Dr. Alzheimer's object test)

- Complete medical history

- Blood and other tests to rule out other possible causes

- Brain scans

Extensive research, however, is underway to develop a reliable blood test to make the diagnosis possible. In doing so, physicians will then be able to screen more people for the devastating illness, thus allowing quicker and improved therapies to slow the disease's progression. As our population continues to age, the race to find a cure and more effective treatments grows more significant. Researchers continue to voice alarm that the number of people with Alzheimer's and the number that will get it soon is rising dramatically.

HOW IS ALZHEIMER'S LINKED TO DIABETES?

For some time, scientists and physicians have known of the increased risk of Alzheimer's disease in people with diabetes – by as much as 65%. The reasons why have mystified researchers, while sparking some hope that a link between the two diseases would help to treat one or both.

Thus, the first steps in a potential breakthrough in the understanding of Alzheimer's disease through a link to diabetes highlighted the Tenth International Conference on Alzheimer's and Related Disorders in the summer of 2006.

Several research studies, reported at the conference, speculated that insulin deficient or resistant cells cut off vital blood sugar to brain neurons thus disabling the ability to remove clumps of incapacitating Alzheimer's amyloid. Other studies pointed to a more complex interaction that begins with the destruction of a brain cell's energy "factories" due to lack of usable glucose.

The most tantalizing of this research centers on the very recent discovery that insulin is produced in the brain as well as the pancreas. Building on that foundation, a team of researchers at Brown Medical School demonstrated that Alzheimer's is a brain-specific disorder similar to Type 1 and 2 diabetes, though differing in its most profound consequences. Led by a Dr. Suzanne de la Monte, the Brown team discovered that insulin receptors in the brain begin to disappear early in the onset of Alzheimer's and continue to decline as the disease progresses. Because of these findings, the Brown Team is recommending the use of Type 3 Diabetes to describe Alzheimer's.

These researchers also were able to replicate Alzheimer's in rats by injecting a compound know to destroy insulin producing cells and cause diabetes. The affected rat brains displayed the same plaque deposits, neurofibrillary tangles and diminished size found in human Alzheimer's patients.

In the September 2006 issue of the Journal of Alzheimer's Disease, the same team reported the first set of findings to indicate that Alzheimer's patients could be treated in early stages of the disease by stimulating a brain receptor that controls insulin responses. In this new study, scientists were able to diminish or even halt the progression of Alzheimer's disease through the use of compounds already, or on track to be, approved by the FDA for treatment of Type 2 diabetes.

Dr. de la Monte noted, "This raises the possibility that you can treat patients with mild cognitive impairment who have possible or probable Alzheimer's disease. This is really amazing because right now there's just no treatment that works."[2]

It is hard to overstate the potential of these discoveries for people suffering from diabetes, Alzheimer's or both.

[Note: as of this printing, only small fragments of the research linking Alzheimer's and diabetes is published and available. Additional content will be included in later printings as well as on the website: www.type4diabetes.com.]

In Addition

■ Read

- Nancy L Mace and Peter V. Rabins, <u>36-Hour Day</u> (New York, NY: Warner, rev. 2001)

- Joanne Koenig Coste and Robert Butler, <u>Learning to Speak Alzheimer's</u> (Houghton Mifflin, 2004)

■ Search

- <u>Alzheimer's Association</u> < http://www.alz.org/>.

- <u>Alzheimer's Foundation of America</u> < http://www.alzfdn.org/>.

■ Endnotes

1. "Alzheimer's Disease," <u>NIH Senior Health</u> January 2005, < http://nihseniorhealth.gov/alzheimersdisease/toc.html>.

2. "Insulin receptor stops progression of Alzheimer's disease," <u>Journal of Alzheimer's Disease</u>, September 2006 < http://www. j-alz.com/press/2006/2006092101.html>.

You can locate updated information
and additional links by visiting:
www.type4diabetes.com.

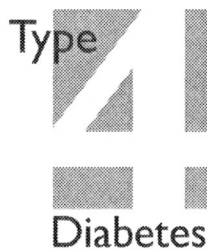

Type 4
Diabetes

Chapter 7

- Blood Sugar Testing

- Home Glucose Meters

Chapter 7
The Importance of Testing

From the beginning of my journey I accepted the value of a testing meter, geeky toy or not. If I polled everyone I know with diabetes, I could easily divide them into two groups. Those who carry a determination to manage, control or even conquer the disease some day swear by the daily use of a meter. The other group of "I'll take my meds and get by" avoid glucose testing except for those infrequent visits to the doctor to renew a prescription.

Granted that there are valid reasons for not needing to, wanting to or being able to test several times each week, if not each day. No doubt the reasons exist; I just don't agree. Yes, we know so much more then we did just 10 to 15 years ago about diabetes and the broader category of glucose metabolism problems. And, yes, people with diabetes and related disorders are so much more fortunate today than at any time previous.

The reality is, however, that for all of the research poured into glucose metabolism issues by the government, research institutes and the pharmaceutical industry, we survive with more questions unanswered than answered. Each person unfortunate enough to have diabetes and related disorders can make a difference and help move us closer to more answers by taking the time to help himself or herself through persistent and consistent meter use.

TEST. TRACK. TRANSFER.

Test whenever you are not sure of your glucose level. Track the results automatically with a meter that stores 200-500 tests or use a simple logbook and a pencil. Transfer the test results to your doctor on a regular basis. There simply is no such reality as too much data and information.

Implicitly, I understood that concept from the beginning. Accept, for the moment, that this understanding was driven by my quirky personality traits of being more curious than most. Granted. Now, however, the basis for my unshakable belief in "Test, Track and Transfer" resides in the incredible, life-changing outcome of my own testing.

You do not have to be a nerd, geek or techie to make this work. Paper logbooks come with most meters. Read and record the test result in the logbook each time. Then take the time periodically to review the results and see if patterns show up. That is the point where I reached the amazing fork in my journey.

Prior to the glucose testing, daily logging already occupied a part of my day. Given a regimen of 10-12 medications a day with varying doses, I had to keep track of the ups and downs of my life with autonomic neuropathy. If a day turned out particularly bad with a high level of pain, diarrhea and severe mental fatigue, I needed to know the events that led up to it. Did I not get enough sleep? Did I walk too far? Did I try to do too much around the house or during the limited hours I worked? What medications did I take to ease the pain and what were the results?

Even more, I wanted to know what led up to the good days with less pain and fewer problems. How did I feel after a combination of meds? If I felt better, for how long would it last? Do I need to take more frequent breaks during the day? Do I need to wait more than one day between longer walks?

Being a persistent emailer even on the feeling bad days, I found little work in jotting an electronic note to myself in a text file. Truly, it helped. Autonomic neuropathy is not well understood. The best specialists only can give you some guidance that may or may not work for a specific individual. Add a mouthful of meds and it's a best guess situation. Tracking is the only way, unless you want to be a victim and just suffer along. Not me, thank you.

My diary for autonomic neuropathy existed. Adding a tracking diary for glucose tests? Not a big deal at all.

Software for tracking varies in quality, ease of use and cost, some details of which are provided later in this chapter. I started by using the monitoring software sold by LifeScan (a Johnson & Johnson company) specifically for its brand of meters. Since it is relatively easy to use with just a small quirk here and there, most people should be able to install and use it (Windows only) in 10-15 minutes. Since I only use Windows computers to check client websites and thrive in a Mac world, I uploaded results to a back-up laptop every 1-2 weeks. Actually, that's more than enough for most people. After all, you do see the individual test result each time on the meter face.

As with any tracking, the importance lies in all of the data that surrounds the actual test. In the case of glucose, you need to track food intake, exercise and other activities that consume energy. Glucose varies in response to energy in (food, drink) and energy out (physical activity). Mental activity also counts in the energy consumption equation since, after all, it is a physical metabolic activity. And don't forget medications, especially those designed for diabetes.

Take for granted that testing and tracking will present you with some surprises— different for everyone. My first surprise, rather shocking admittedly, was how high my glucose soared after some meals. A day lounging on the couch followed by a breakfast the next morning of pancakes and syrup sent my level over 300. To someone dealing with diabetes for more than a few years, the 300-level is not outlandish. Been there, done that, right?

Not to me, though. I started seeing results in the 200-

300 levels often in the first months after I first learned that I suffered from, at least, prediabetes. My numbers should not have been anywhere near this level. Not if the diabetes, if the glucose metabolism problem, was just beginning. But, if the diabetes had been a problem for some time, why had it not been noticed in early blood tests?

As I complete this book, I now have a reasonable theory: the night before a quarterly blood test for tolerance to neuropathy medications, I tended to load up on food (mostly carbs) just before bedtime since breakfast was going to be much later than normal. Given what I have discerned to be my typical pattern, a load of carbs late at night is likely to send my glucose level soaring and then crashing. By the time I arrived for the blood test, my "numbers looked good." In fact, these earlier blood tests took a "snapshot" at the wrong time.

The past is the past. The focus needs to be on keeping the glucose levels within acceptable ranges. From Dr. Peter's book, and other excellent resources, I had already knew about important studies in the UK and the US related to managing Type 2 without medications — through regular exercise and a controlled diet. A bell went off with those high numbers and my focus turned to food and activity, quickly and with determination. I can, I will bring down those numbers.

Exercise, unfortunately, presents frequent obstacles and stumbling points for people with autonomic neuropathy. There are issues with heart rate, blood pressure, duration and frequency that vary from individual to individual, and even from day to day with the same person. Additionally, many people with neuropathy must contend with temperature intolerance and a limited ability to sweat. Even patients suffering from the worst cases of autonomic neuropathy will likely benefit from some exercise. But, when you face all of the side effects that accompany exercise, just lying on the couch is so tempting.

Limiting calories and carbs, or at least switching to more complex carbohydrates, is an easier task for most people with autonomic neuropathy, but not always as simple as it might seem. Misfiring nerve cells, not the actual diet, can lead to those charming charges to the bathroom. A large meal may end with little time to be broken down in your system, so you end up not getting enough calories. Even if the previous meal remains, bouts of nausea will change what you want to eat. A comfortable bowl of mac and cheese often rates higher on the desirability level than the healthier salmon on greens.

Regardless of the obstacles, I made a resolute pact with myself early into the fall of 2005 that the level of exercise was going up considerably, as was the nutritional quality of food, while the total quantity of food was going to go down. Sheer determination to get the glucose levels down overrode many of the neuropathic obstacles.

Yes, the pain did increase along with other discomforts. No, I didn't increase any of my medications. Rather, I turned to massage and acupuncture to alleviate as much pain as possible. Those two therapies helped, fortunately.

Believe in the results and recommendations of the diabetes prevention studies. I do. Within weeks, the glucose number showed significant improvement. Highs above 200 became infrequent. I was eating better and exercising more. But, as expected, the problems with neuropathy increased as well.

Seeing positive changes with my glucose levels proved to be all the motivation I needed to keep going. Having to deal with additional nerve discomfort prompted increased attention to my daily tracking. I needed to learn more about my changing lifestyle and manage it with even more determination.

In Detail

SHOULD I USE A BLOOD GLUCOSE METER?

Wondrous in its capabilities, the home glucose meter revolutionized diabetes management beginning in 1980. No longer would a trip to the doctor's office or hospital be required to test blood sugar levels. Given that your glucose level changes constantly throughout the day and night, the handheld device finally provided the information necessary for doctors and their patients to gain meaningful control: not too high and not too low.

Though the meters quickly became popular with Type 1 patients, many in the medical community initially opposed their use arguing that: 1) laboratory tests are inherently more accurate, and 2) patients should not be left on their own to interpret those results. As meters continue to improve the ease of use and test accuracy, those arguments have abated, but not ceased entirely.

True, home testing meters cannot obtain, today, the accuracy of a laboratory test. Most meters, in fact, are considered to be "accurate enough" if a test result is within 20% of a laboratory test of the same blood sample. When testing for "highs" this level of precision is considered adequate. For example, if your glucose is a true 250 mg/dl in a standard laboratory test, your home meter could display a reading between 200-300. Although that is a large range, every number in that range indicates a higher than acceptable level of glucose. In actual use, many meters display numbers much closer to the test standard than the allowable 20%. And, manufacturers are working to improve those results.

On the low blood sugar side (hypoglycemia), current meters offer less satisfying results for the 20% differential. For example, the difference between 72-48 (60 +/- 20%) is very significant in managing hypoglycemia. For more discussion on low blood sugar and meters, please read Chapter 9.

The reluctance of physicians to recommend home testing for Type 2 patients appears on the wane. Many published physician/authors, in fact, state that all of their patients now are required to test at home and to track the results on paper or through the built-in memory storage of numerous meters. And, why not? Giving a patient a critical tool that can be used to better control a serious illness just seems obvious beyond an argument to me.

In the time before home meters, no practical way existed for patients to understand how diet, exercise and stress impacted blood sugar levels. Knowing what a fasting glucose level is on the one day each quarter when you visit your doctor just isn't good enough.

The importance of a meter and home testing comes from observing your blood glucose levels over time and under different lifestyle situations — not a specific test result. If you are concerned about the accuracy of your meter, bring it along when you visit your doctor for the next lab test. At the same time blood is drawn out of your arm, take a meter test and note the result. Compare that with the lab result in a few days.

HOW DO I CHOOSE A METER?

As a practical manner, you may not have much of a choice if your doctor requires the use of a specific brand or model. And, your insurance company may be just as limiting. The latter restriction is based on cost control. The doctor's requirement may have more to do with standardizing computer tracking software in the medical office.

Left on your own, publications such as *Diabetes Forecast* and *Diabetes Health*, publish annual reports as well as frequent website updates. Pick up a copy of either and you'll also see plenty of ads from the companies that manufacture meters. Comparison articles also can be found in *Consumer's Reports* and similar magazines/websites.

For reasons having to do with tracking software (see Chapter 8), I strongly recommend four brands of meters:

- Accu-Chek (made by Roche Diagnostics)[1]

- Ascensia (Bayer HealthCare)[2]

- Freestyle (Abbott Diabetes Care)[3]

- OneTouch (LifeScan/Johnson&Johnson)[4]

Most glucose meters are actually comprised of three items that are similar from manufacturer to manufacturer:

1. The battery-powered meter (typically about the size and shape of a stop watch or 'fat' flip-style cell phone)

2. Test strips (about 1" long and a ¼-inch wide)

3. Lancing (finger pricking) device

Strips are kept in a closed container and inserted into the meter at the time of a test. After pricking your finger (or forearm), you position the attached strip into the blood droplet and wait 5-20 seconds for the result to be displayed on the LCD screen. How the meter actually performs the analysis requires a strong background in biochemistry. Suffice to say that the glucose in your blood reacts with dried chemicals on the strip to permit great or lesser amounts of battery current to flow through the strip.

Given the rapidly growing demand for meters, leading manufacturers constantly seek an "edge" in one brand over another, despite the fact that the chemistry and physics are the same. Some models eliminate the need for inserting individual test strips, relying on a drum or disc preloaded with 10 or more strips. These devices, along with some individual strips, eliminate the need for "coding" the meter for each vial of purchased strips.

On the devices that have to be coded, you enter the number on the outside of each vial of strips you open. The reason for the coding is to assist in making the combination of strips and meter as accurate as possible. As the strips are made, patches are tested for accuracy and the results of those tests used to determine the proper meter code. This allows companies to simplify the manufacturing process and lessen the need to toss out less accurate batches.

The lancing devices are similar in size and feel similar to a thick ballpoint pen. On the "business end" you insert a small, sterilized pin, push back on the spring, hold it against a finger (or forearm) and press the spring release. Despite advertising claims, most of the time it does sting a little. One company even refers to its brand of lancets as "ultrasoft." As if! Expect a little pain since your finger trips are loaded with nerve endings. For that reason, some people prefer to test on their forearms where fewer nerve endings are found.

I tend to bruise easily so I find the forearm testing less appealing even if it is less likely to hurt. What I have found, though, is that the Accu-Chek Multiclix[5] lancing device, with its preloaded drum of six lancets, is the least annoying in the pain department. I use it with a LifeScan UltraOne Touch Smart meter and find the overall experience to be simple and accurate.

WHAT ABOUT THE A I C TEST?

Every 3-6 months, your doctor likely will recommend that you come in for a glycated hemoglobin blood test. Avoiding the pain of biochemistry once again, this test measures the average amount of glucose in your red blood cells in the previous 90-120 days. The test result comes back as a percentage. By comparing it to your meter readings, you can gauge how well, on average, you maintained a good glucose level over the last few months.

TABLE 7-1	Comparing A1C to Blood Glucose Tests		
A1C (%)	Ave. Glucose (mg/dL)	Ave. Glucose (mmol/L)	Comment
4-5.9	< 120	< 6.7	Considered normal
6	120	6.7	Above this, generally prediabetes.
7	150	8.3	Above this, generally diabetes. Target for people with diabetes is 7 or below.
>8	>180	>10.0	Unhealthy

An A1C offers a valuable "check" on your daily meter readings and record keeping. It should not be considered as a replacement for meter readings since it is an average. Quarterly A1C tests will not give you sufficient information upon which to base a healthy diet and exercise plan — especially for those with Type 4 symptoms.

In Addition

To learn more about diabetes testing:

■ Read

- "2007 Resource Guide," <u>Diabetes Forecast</u>, January 2007.

■ Search

- "Glucose Meters and Diabetes Management," <u>US Food and Drug Administration</u> < http://www.fda.gov/diabetes/glucose. html>.

- "Meters & Pumps," <u>DiabetesHealth</u> < http://www.diabeteshealth.com/browse,3001.html>.

- "Diabetes Technology," <u>DiabetesMall</u> < http://www.diabetesnet.com/diabetes_technology/blood_glucose_meters.php>.

- "Blood-Glucose Monitors," <u>Consumer Reports</u> < http://www.consumerreports.org>.

■ Endnotes

1. <u>Accu-Chek</u> <http://www.accu-chek.com>.

2. <u>Ascensia</u> <http://www.ascensia.com>.

3. <u>Abbott Diabetes Care</u> < http://abbottdiabetescare.com/>.

4. <u>LifeScan</u> < http://www.lifescan.com/>.

5. <u>Accu-Chek</u> < http://www.accu-chek.com/us/rewrite/content/en_US/2.1.6.1:10/article/ACCM_general_article_2836. htm?SOURCE=GOOG%26KEYWORD%3Dp>.

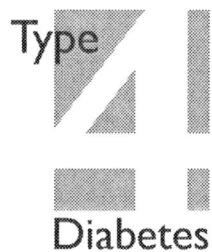

Type

Diabetes

Chapter 8

- Testing & Tracking

- Glucose Tracking Software

Chapter 8
The Breakthrough

When does something useful become inspired? What makes an idea a breakthrough? My guess falls back to constant searching and luck. Dedicating myself to constant activity and armed with more than my share of luck, the fall of 2005 proved productive in the breakthrough category.

As the testing and tracking continued in parallel with the ongoing diary on neuropathy, I had reason to focus on both, although separately. The high glucose numbers kept going down. Good. But, as the highs came down I began to pay attention to the low end, the fasting number, and how the glucose level responded downward after certain food and exercise combinations. Curious data, but at the time, not significant to me.

Turning to the issue of my chronically faulty nerves, I paid considerable attention to the events surrounding good days and bad days. More exercise meant new patterns to observe. Now, though, I started to focus more closely on events and how I felt at different times of the day. How did I feel waking up? How did I feel later in the morning? How about the afternoon? Any patterns?

Call it luck, perspiration or inspiration. I kept looking at the notes for one disease and then the other. I created a few graphs and charts (nerd, remember?). I kept looking back and forth at the two separate groups until I started seeing two as one. One person. Me. Two different problems. Could they be two related problems? Well … maybe … perhaps… Yes, two related problems in the one person.

The first pattern. If my post-breakfast glucose was higher than the fasting number, the day tended to be "good" on the neuropathy front. Higher post-meal glucose is the expected result for healthy people as well as those with diabetes.

Second pattern. If the post-breakfast reading was the same as before breakfast then I tended to have a so-so day. Part of the day good and part of it not as good.

Third pattern. If post-meal glucose was lower than fasting — certainly not the expected result — then the day was going to be a real pain, literally and figuratively.

Fourth pattern. The home run. The lower the post-meal glucose relative to the pre-breakfast reading, the more likely I was to experience a higher level of pain.

In a later chapter, I am going to discuss in more depth carbohydrate-sensitive (reactive) hypoglycemia and the lower glucose response that some people have to eating certain foods — specifically those high in simple carbohydrates — as well as certain medications. It is not a normal reaction, but it does happen in some people. And, it is not completely understood. More importantly, the consequences of reactive hypoglycemia are also not well known and frequently dismissed by some in the medical community as trivial or, worse, non-existent.

I, however, experienced the lower glucose response on a frequent basis with non-trivial, quite real consequences. What did that mean to me? How should I respond to this information? Only one thing appeared certain. I had journeyed into unchartered territory. None of the books and none of Google searches yielded much guidance. On my own.

Three major events dominated my journey in the weeks that followed the beginning of testing and tracking. Discovering the patterns came first. It may seem obvious in retrospect, but I thought for many days about the significance of the discovery and just couldn't make the logic leap to the next step. On days when my post breakfast glucose goes down, pain awaits. So, what do I do about it?

The large diabetes community deserves enormous credit for making amazing inroads into the American mind-set. No doubt, most diabetes educators, physicians and related healt care providers anxiously seek even higher level of awareness and action. But, considering how quickly we have emerged from the days of whispers about the "spilling" disease to a weekly program on cable giant CNBC, many deserve hearty congratulations. Aware people do think — even if they take little or no action — about the dangers of elevated blood sugar.

Not so regarding the downside — low blood sugar. In the 1970s low blood sugar, hypoglycemia became a topic of great popular interest with the publication of a few books on the topic.   Suddenly lots of people flocked to doctors certain that their medical problems had hypoglycemia as the root cause. To detractors, hypoglycemia quickly became a "fad" disease. How unfortunate, but understandable. With only limited lab tests available to test glucose levels, even getting a good handle on a specific patient's changing glucose levels was all but impossible.

The concept that low blood sugar levels could cause significant problem for people not using insulin soon garnered much derision within the medical community. An idea that arose quickly was cast aside almost as fast. People with real problems were left without a good answer to the question, "Why do I feel lousy?" The same question I asked three decades later.

Now these thoughts ran through my brain:
Dummy! Raise your glucose level.
Should I? How? Risks? Help!
Forget the help. Who is going to believe me? Risks. Well, if I elevate my glucose too much, I could hasten the day when high blood sugar problems are my primary concern. How. Diabetes patients know well the routine for elevating blood sugar when it gets dangerously low due to insulin or oral medications.

Fruit juice. Hard candy. Glucose tablets. It all came down to, "Should I"?

Right after Thanksgiving 2005, I began to take 4-gram glucose tablets between 9-10 am every morning that post-breakfast glucose strayed lower than my fasting level. I opted for glucose tablets because I could control the amount of glucose with some accuracy. Actually, I couldn't find a formula for elevating glucose levels with Belgian chocolate. If I had …

Also, glucose tablets are cheap. Ten to 20 cents each from most drug, food and discount stores. Quickly dissolving, they should increase your blood sugar level within 10 minutes or so. So, I would test again until my glucose reached the target level of 100. Still low? Dissolve another tablet.

It is time to bring up the topic of the glucose target level. And, with this discussion will come lots of derision from medical experts. The safest bet I could wager today is that nine out of every 10 medical doctors dismiss the notion that any real low blood sugar symptoms occur with readings in the 90-100 range. Definitely at 50. Maybe 60. Hardly at 70. Above that? It's fantasy. It's in his head.

The chorus of nay-sayers constitutes a very broad segment of the health care community. But, not all. "My experience leads me to conclude that there is, in fact, a reaction to sudden increases and falls in blood sugar levels. This may be due to too much insulin released, although it could be due to other hormones released by the stomach and other organs as well," notes Dr. Peters in addressing the lack of substantive information about the consequences of low blood sugar.[1]

"The shakiness and blurred vision is not necessarily due to actual low blood sugar levels. More likely they relate to the fact that blood sugar levels are falling. This is not science [her emphasis] — just my personal observation (and the observation of many others." [2]

Frankly, I didn't care a bit about commonly-accepted medical "facts". I established the 100 level from my own fairly scientific studies. The glucose meter I use is accurate, reliable and scientific. Sure, self-observed symptoms are highly subjective, but totally valid to me.

The in-your-face reality about the 100 level is that it worked. On those days with post-breakfast lows, when I pushed the number to 100 or above, the level, frequency and duration of pain and related neuropathic problems decreased. Now, I had some sense of control. And that was a very empowering feeling.

Next step. Positively influence the impact of my neuropathy symptoms for 12-24 hours. Within a few weeks, that wonderful goal had been achieved.

Thinking back on those December days when it I reached this plateau, honestly, I believed I reached the ultimate step: some control influence. I never, ever expected that total control lay just around the corner — and one fortuitous mistake away.

In Detail

TRACKING AND ANALYZING. SOFTWARE. BODY JOURNAL.

Data alone are useless. Only when you start to place it into context, study and analyze it do the data become useful. It turns into information. So it is with all those readings from your glucose meter. Bravo for being committed, buying a meter, learning how to use it and then going through the lancing and testing on a regular basis. But, if you don't work with those readings, then why go through all of that effort?

TEST. TRACK. TRANSFER.

The 2nd step is tracking. It's great to start with the paper logbook that comes with every meter. Note the time of the day, the test results and make some quick notes about your life at the time: before breakfast, after a meal, the food you ate, the time and intensity of exercise, your stress level. Only a very select few can remember all of these daily events a few days from now. So write it down.

Keep looking back from time to time to see if you can determine a few patterns. Look for trends, identify oddities that make you wonder. Take notes. Ask yourself questions. Keep testing. Keep tracking and analyzing.

WHAT ABOUT TRACKING RESULTS WITH SOFTWARE?

An easy question for any geek. Of course! Some people work to live. Others live to work. We live to compute!

For the sane world, however, the question of using a

computer program to track and analyze results offers no pat answer. If you basically tolerate computers as a necessary nuisance, or even hate them, then don't add this burden to the testing routine. It will only make you less likely to keep to a regular schedule of testing. If you feel comfortable using a computer to send email and do some Web surfing, then you'll find computer tracking to be simple enough and well worth the time and effort.

First, make sure that you purchase a meter such as the OneTouch Ultra or Onetouch UltraSmart. These meters, along with many others from leading companies, have a data port on the side. You could, of course, use any simple meter and manually enter the test results via a keyboard. But, why not make life simpler and let the computers talk to each other?

You connect the meter to your computer (usually with a special USB cable). Launch your software application program and follow the instructions for uploading from the meter to your computer. You will probably have to purchase the cable separately for $15-$30. For that price, you often get a software tracking application, though some companies give you the software for free.

WHICH SOFTWARE APPLICATION SHOULD I USE?

The tracking applications that come from the meter companies certainly do the job and they are a good place to start — especially if the software comes with the meter or is available as a free download. As with the meter, some doctors require the use of a specific program so check with your doctor first. After all the third part of the essential command is to "Transfer" your information to a physician or diabetes educator.

In my early testing and tracking, I used the OneTouch Diabetes Management software. The user interface is a bit basic and some of the commands seem quirky, but it does work as advertised.

You also have a choice of software from third-party developers with lots of extra features. If you are a Mac person, your path is clear: as of this writing all of the meter-specific software are Windows-only.

HealthEngage[3] offers a diabetes-tracking program that works with the Windows, Mac and Linux operating systems as well as with Palm, PocketPC devices and iPod devices. Prices start at $60. The program is solid and works with FreeStyle and OneTouch meters. The company offers similar programs for tracking many other chronic illnesses as well as diet and exercise.

The grand prize for tracking software, though, goes to The Body Journal[4]. Located in Toronto, the company's flagship product ranks among the most elegant, sophisticated yet easy to understand and use consumer applications that I tested — and I see a lot. At $49 (US), the program is a one-stop home and personal medical filing cabinet. Family medical records, emergency contacts, medications, daily exercise and food logs all come together in this one application. You can track glucose as well as dozens of other home and laboratory tests. You can purchase form the company directly or through Amazon.com.

The Body Journal also offers you the advantage of backing up your information to its computers for safekeeping. Your data is password protected, but remember nothing is totally secure. I have found no reason to question the security of my information on their computers, however, and welcome the built-in backup capability.

The numerous reports and graphs can be viewed locally or sent to your doctor via email.

If you are using a computer to track, at least download and test this program. It's worth the time.

In Addition

■ Search

- "Diabetes Software," <u>DiabetesMall</u> 2005 < http://www.diabe-tesnet.com/diabetes_technology/software.php>.

- [Note: unfortunately, as of this printing, information and reviews about diabetes testing and tracking software is very limited. Most the sites that appear through searches appear to have not been updated for years. Hopefully this will change in the near future. If you have an opinion on software and wish to share it, please visit: www.Type4Diabetes.com. Thanks.}

■ Endnotes

1. Anne Peters, <u>Conquering Diabetes</u> (New York: Hudson Street Press, 2005) p. 65

2. Peters, p. 67

3. "HealthEngage Diabetes 3.8," <u>HealthEngage</u> < http://www.healthengage.com/healthengagediabetes.html>.

4. <u>The Body Journal</u> < http://www.bodyjournal.com/>.

    You can locate updated information
    and additional links by visiting:
    www.type4diabetes.com.

Type Diabetes

Chapter 9

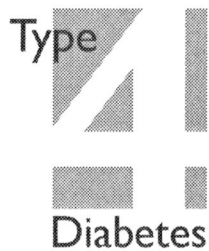

■ Hypoglycemia

Chapter 9
The Curtain Goes Up

Women really do have an advantage or two in the accessories area. They can get away with carrying a purse. American men, on the other hand, shove a wallet into one back pocket, drop keys in one front pocket, change in the other and hang the cell phone on a belt. It's ugly, inconvenient and hurts. Truly. But, we keep doing what our fathers did and our sons imitate us.

You can forget social norms, though, when you are on a routine of a dozen medications a day and actually leave home. The pharmacy must come with you. And, unless you want to bring the male equivalent of a purse or the just-as-messy laptop case with you, what's a guy to do with all those prescriptions?

My travel companions. For pain: Bufferin, Tylenol, Frova, Imitrex tablets and an Imitrex pen injector for treating increasing levels of raw discomfort. Neurontin twice a day to ward off some of the pain. Effexor to assist in managing two neurotransmitters: serotonin and norepinephrine. Migre-lief, an herbal-based medication popular in German to treat headaches. Coreg, a beta-blocker, to assist in proper heart function. Klonopin to treat abnormal neurological activity. Propantheline to control the sudden attacks of diarrhea. Oh, and Levoxyl, since I don't have a thyroid gland.

Short of wearing farmer's overalls, no men's pant pocket can hold all of these even if I just sort them out into one of those snappy "daily med-minders." So, I had my excuse for a male travel bag. And, it worked well for the wallet, keys, cell phone and the occasional camera.

On the not-so-frequent trips away from home, the travel case became essential out of simple fear that putting all of meds into the suitcase was a sure way to tempt fate, baggage handlers and the wonderful world of post-9/11 security. You live by the pill and fear dying without them.

Armed with this travel case, James and I went to New York City for the holiday period between Christmas and New Year's in 2005. Call me sentimental, but growing up in the New York suburbs, Christmas would not be Christmas without a trip to see the lights at Rockefeller Center. I'm grown now, so a Broadway performance and shopping at Macy's always makes it onto the trip agenda. Though the neuropathy limited the shopping time at Herald Square to usually one floor and an item or two.

On the evening of December 28, we sat down in "we-can-only-afford-these-once-a-year" seats for a performance of *Avenue Q*. After a hectic day of travel, at least for me, I longed for an enjoyable evening filled with laughs and some already memorable songs my two grown children had played over and over for me. Just as the curtain was going up, the awful sensation that words cannot adequately express erupted in my head.

The signal always means an autonomic neuropathy attack is moments away. The pain is coming plus a heaping helping of nasty disorders. The quicker and stronger the signal, the more misery I will experience. Unless I act fast, I can be sure that I am mere moments away from some quality time in the closest restroom. Please, may one be near by!

Have no fear, I told myself as I have over and over again. You'll have to grit through some of the pain, but at least the other symptoms can be managed with a few more pills. Right here in the male purse.

Uh, oh. Actually, the words were much stronger than

that! I had emptied the case at the apartment we were borrowing from friends so I could leave the non-essentials behind for the evening. Interrupted by a call, I never completed the task.

This just can't be happening. It's not fair!

Knowing it to be an exercise in futility I dumped the keys, phone, wallet, breathe mints and other odds and ends in my lap — to the chagrin of people around me — desperate to discover a random pill or two. Nothing. Except for a small package of glucose tablets that somehow remained stuck inside during the aborted house cleaning. Little good they'll do, I thought sullenly as I looked for the nearest exit sign.

Desperation is the real mother of invention. With nothing else to do, I started to rationalize that if the glucose tablets could help improve my bad days, maybe it would have some impact right now as an attack loomed. Well, it couldn't hurt, I concluded as I chewed on all four tablets. Then I sat back prepping myself for the onrushing attack.

It never came.

Trying to focus on the show to manage as much of the forecast pain as possible, I soon jerked my head in one of those moments when you realize something is really wrong. Except that it was really right. I didn't feel anything. No pain. No abdominal swelling. No leg cramps. No blurry vision. No tingling. No dizziness. Nothing.

"Wow!", I finally exclaimed out loud after a few amazing minutes of no symptoms. Unfortunately, this moment came at a very quiet point in the show and I am sure that some of the folks around me didn't appreciate my sudden utterance. But, I didn't care. I got a "please behave" look from my partner and I whispered back some assurance about "wait until I tell you this at intermission."

Forget the ending of the musical. The star of the night was four small, sweet glucose tablets. Outstanding performance. Worthy of a Tony right then and there. For a "nothing performance." The attack never came. Not that evening. And when another attack started up the next day, I slammed back some more glucose. A repeat performance. Encore, encore.

Actually, I thought it too good to be true. "Must be a fluke," I told myself each time the glucose treatment worked to thwart an impending attack. It just couldn't be a real solution. For the next three weeks I kept even tighter track of glucose levels and my overall health, the level of pain, etc. When the end of January rolled around and I had been free of autonomic neuropathy attacks for more than five weeks, euphoria set in.

Call me overly dramatic or whatever, but I cannot over-state how much this discovery meant to me. Only those who have dealt with chronic, persistent, constant pain for year after year totally understand how that crushing weight of pain im-pacts each day. When it suddenly disappears, your life begins anew. You realize how much effort it took each and every day to get through and cope with the pain as you attempt to live as fully as possible. It is exhausting. And, now I now longer had to deal with that work.

Freedom. Exhilaration. Confidence. Confusion. Annoy-ance. Anger.

Why did I go through six years of misery? Why didn't my doctors know about this? Why didn't they tell me? This is insane. How could a non-medical person such as myself stumble on to this? Am I crazy? Well, debatable perhaps, but besides the point.

Test. Track. Transfer. Time now for the first part of that formula. I wrote down everything I could about my experiences, added charts and graphs and sent copies to my three main doc-tors. To say that I was met with skepticism is an intense under-statement. Even from my doctors, the response could best be described as dismissive. "Please! Get real, Bob. Not possible. It's just a momentary thing. You'll feel crappy again soon enough. "

Thanks for the confidence and the good wishes. How-ever, one issue was resolved in my head. If my doctors didn't know about a link between a 90-100 level glucose reading being considered low and autonomic neuropathy, then I doubted that many in the medical world knew. OK, I am not angry at my doctors for not telling me. But, what is going on?

Rejected by my own doctors, the only thing to do was to keep going with my own treatment, test and track as never before, and dive into research to see if anyone might know.

On the research front, I discovered a few tantalizing tidbits of information, some very frustrating citations and not much more. Prior to all of this, I had not read the sections in Dr. Peters' book on hypoglycemia since it "didn't apply to me." Now I read those sections over and over again with a sense that someone does know, or at least has a hint, a sixth sense that lots more about low blood glucose needs to be investigated. Dr. Peters' book offered me some comfort, but also a renewed sense of living in a dream. I may be smart, some may say arrogant, but come on. How could I expect to have "discovered" this link?

Driven by the determination to avoid a return to pain, and with a lot of trepidation, I pushed along further on the journey.

In Detail

Hypoglycemia. Within the medical community about the only consensus possible is on how to spell the word; everything else is subject to debate. More than a few physicians, in fact, doubt its very existence. And, many more don't accept it as a condition except for people with diabetes who mismanage insulin and/or oral medications.

The state of denial concerning hypoglycemia is understandable although very, very frustrating — and potential harmful for millions of people.

Detractors frequently point to the 1960s when hypoglycemia emerged as a "in vogue" disorder — especially for women. Patients flocked to doctors offices with complaints about "feeling low," light-headedness and nervousness. Label it hypoglycemia, prescribe some diet changes and send the patient home. Such became the route for many people and their doctors. Oral glucose tolerance tests frequently supplied supportive data.

Upon further investigation, some researchers concluded that the glucose tolerance tests "proved" that the condition was all "in the mind." Women in the studies were given the tests without learning of their blood sugar levels. Rather, the researchers just asked for symptoms before and after the glucose tolerance test. When no obvious correlation between actual levels and symptoms was observed in many cases, the conclusion pointed to hypoglycemia being a "fad" and not real.

Absent the need, or money, to delve further into the issue, these studies became the rule of evidence and large segments of the medical community turned away from considering or treating hypoglycemia – except for people with insulin-treated diabetes.

WHAT IS HYPOGLYCEMIA?

The US government's National Diabetes Information Clearinghouse (NDIC) offers the simple definition: "Hypoglycemia, also called low blood sugar, occurs when your blood glucose (blood sugar) level drops too low to provide enough energy for your body's activities."[1]

Symptoms of hypoglycemia include:

- Hunger

- Nervousness and shakiness

- Perspiration

- Dizziness or light-headedness

- Sleepiness

- Confusion

- Difficulty speaking

- Feeling anxious or weak

Hypoglycemia can also occur while you are asleep with symptoms such as:

- Crying out or having nightmares

- Finding that your pajamas or sheets are damp from perspiration

- Feeling tired, irritable or confused when you wake

A blood glucose reading of 70 mg/dl (3.9 mmo/l) is frequently used as the point where hypoglycemia symptoms occur. As readings fall, the symptoms are generally considered to become worse. These conclusions belie the fact that "normal" blood glucose varies with age, population groups and circumstances. Slowly gaining support within the medical community is the conclusion that hypoglycemic symptoms can occur at much higher glucose levels; more the result of how rapidly glucose drops rather than the actual level.

As one physician noted to me, "it's really common sense to accept that a diabetic who has spent months with glucose levels in the 300's is going to experience symptoms of hypoglycemia when glucose levels drop to 150 or so."

Why then, I asked, do you read in book after book, article after article — written my doctors and other medical experts — that symptoms of hypoglycemia cannot happen above 70 or so? "Dogma," he replied. "You learn something in med school and it just becomes a rote response."

Hopefully, at least, some of that dogma is about to be changed,

THE DOWNSIDE OF FAULTY GLUCOSE METABOLISM

Glucose, a form of sugar, is a critical fuel your body needs. Carbohydrates are the main dietary source of glucose. Key sources of carbs are:

- Potatoes

- Bread

- Rice

- Tortillas

- Cereal

■ Milk

■ Fruit

■ Table sugar

■ Prepared foods rich in sugars

During the digestion process, the carbs are broken down into glucose that is then absorbed into your bloodstream and carried to your cells. Glucose, however, requires a specific hormone to enter the cells where it is used as energy. That hormone is insulin either produced by your pancreas or injected in people with diabetes.

When you produce more glucose than you need (by eating too many carbs), your body stores the extra glucose in your liver, muscles and fat as glycogen. This "bank account" of stored glucose can then be used as needed when your body requires more fuel.

How does your body signal its need for more fuel? Another hormone produced by the pancreas, glucagon, signals the liver to break down glycogen and release glucose into the blood stream. This balancing act of storing and releasing glucose is essential to balancing blood sugar levels and maintaining your health. When it goes awry, as in diabetes, glucose levels are hard to maintain and can begin to "roller coaster" from too high to too low.

In people treating their diabetes with either insulin or certain oral medications, blood glucose can fall too low for reasons such as:

■ Too little food to digest for glucose (skipping a meal or eating too small a meal)

■ Too much insulin or medication

■ Too much activity of exercise

■ Too much alcohol

People with diabetes using insulin and certain oral drugs attempt to perform the same balancing act in the absence of a healthy internal system. The amount of insulin injected must come close to matching your body's fuel needs and the amount of carbs being ingested. Too much insulin and there is not enough glucose left in the blood to fuel all the cells that need it. Too little insulin and excess glucose begins to build up in the blood. It isn't stored, but rather some of the excess "spills" out through the urine even while damaging smaller vessels.

WHAT ABOUT PEOPLE WHO HAVE NOT BEEN DIAGNOSED WITH DIABETES?

As stated previously, the entire subject of low blood sugar in people without diagnosed diabetes prompts heated discussions within the medical community. A bit of consensus is emerging around two types of hypoglycemia: fasting-related and post-meal.

Fasting Hypoglycemia: linked to certain medications (including large doses of aspirin), alcohol abuse, hormonal deficiencies, certain tumors, critical illnesses and specific conditions that occur in infancy and childhood.

Carbohydrate-Sensitive Hypoglycemia: also called Reactive or Postprandial hypoglycemia, generates the most controversy. As the NDIC notes: "The causes of most cases of reactive hypoglycemia are still open to debate. Some researchers suggest that certain people may be more sensitive to the body's normal release of the hormone epinephrine [more commonly known to the general public as adrenaline], which causes many of the symptoms of hypoglycemia. Others believe that deficiencies in glucagon secretion might lead to hypoglycemia."[2]

Concludes Dr. Peters at USC: "True hypoglycemia, a blood sugar level below 50 mg/dl, may or may not be found in patients with sensitivity to carbohydrates. Because of this physicians have gotten away form calling the feeling of being shaky, hypoglycemia, because it doesn't fit the medical definition for it. **Yet it is a real phenomenon.** [emphasis added] In my experience many people who see me with a diagnosis of newly developed Type 2 diabetes have had this sensitivity for several years. In order to separate this feeling of hypoglycemia from the hypoglycemia that occurs when treating diabetes, I will call it "carbohydrate-sensitive" hypoglycemia, because it is a feeling a low or falling blood sugar after eating carbohydrates."[3]

Dr. R. Paul St. Amand, Assistant Clinical Professor at UCLA School of Medicine, notes: "Hypoglycemia is a word often used to denote a disease when it is actually only a symptom. The term means low blood sugar but often symptoms occur without a particularly low value. This syndrome is better defined as carbohydrate intolerance resulting in symptoms due mainly to an overzealous neuro-endocrine response."[4]

Obviously, more research needs to be done. Too little is known. Too much remains to be gained from a better understanding.

WHAT CAN BE DONE TO PREVENT SYMPTOMS OF HYPOGLYCEMIA?

On this topic, more agreement exists. If you have the hypoglycemic symptoms a concise summary of recommendations includes:

1. Eat 5-6 small meals or snacks each day. By eating smaller meals throughout the day as opposed to the traditional "Big 3," you spread out glucose metabolism and reduce large spikes. Avoid skipping meals.

2. Choose high fiber foods (oat bran nuts, legumes/beans, pears, apples and most veggies)

3. Choose complex carbohydrates over simple ones. Complex carbs (grains, brown rice, oatmeal, fruits, chickpeas, kidney beans) take longer to digest and break down into glucose than simple carbs (sugar, refined flour, white rice).

4. Choose artificial sweeteners such as Splenda. Though derived from sugar, Splenda (sucralose) does not react during metabolism to increase glucose levels.

5. Limit fats.

6. Reduce caffeine. It stimulates the production of adrenaline.

7. Reduce or eliminate alcohol. It contains calories with no nutritional value, and it stimulates insulin levels lowering glucose.

8. Maintain a healthy weight.

9. Exercise regularly. Walking, Yoga, Swimming and T'ai Chi can help you get and stay in shape without undo physical stress.

10. Try consuming a "glucose stabilizing bar" before bedtime, such as ExtendBar.[5] These bars contain slowly-digested cornstarch

and help to maintain glucose levels for up
to nine hours.

In Addition

▪ Read

- Roberta Ruggiero, <u>The Do's and Don'ts of Hypoglycemia</u> (Hollywood, FL: Frederick Fell Publishers, 2004)

- Anita Flegg, <u>Hypoglycemia: The Other Sugar Disease</u> (Ottawa, ON: Book Coach Press, 2005)

- Cheryl Chow and James Chow, <u>Hypoglycemia for Dummies</u> (New York: Wiley, 2003)

▪ Search

- "Hypoglycemia," <u>National Diabetes Information Clearinghouse</u>, March 2003 < http://diabetes.niddk.nih.gov/dm/pubs/hypoglycemia/index.htm>.

- <u>The Hypoglycemia Support Foundation</u> 2006 < http://www.hypoglycemia.org/>.

- "Hypoglycemia," <u>American Diabetes Association</u> 2006 < http://www.diabetes.org/type-2-diabetes/hypoglycemia.jsp>.

▪ Endnotes

1. "Hypoglycemia," National Diabetes Information Clearinghouse < http://diabetes.niddk.nih.gov/dm/pubs/hypoglycemia/index.htm>.

2. "Hypoglycemia"

3. Anne Peters, <u>Conquering Diabetes</u> (New York: Hudson Street Press, 2005) p. 63-64.

4. Paul St. Amand, <u>What Your Doctor May Not Tell You About Fibromyalgia</u> (New York: Warner, 2006)

5. <u>ExtendBar</u> <http://www.extendbar.com>.

You can locate updated information and additional links by visiting: www.type4diabetes.com.

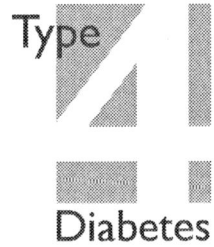

Type
Diabetes

Chapter 10

▪ Insulin-Adrenaline Link

Chapter 10
A New Beginning

I play the lottery every now and then. Yes, I know the odds of winning are minute. So what? Dreams are fun. And, in fact, I did win a car once in a sweepstakes. On my 40th birthday. A red Mazda Miata. What are the odds of that? By the way, you really do not want to win anything unless it comes with enough cash to pay the taxes. Trust me on this one.

So, I accepted the theoretical possibility, although very remote, that I stumbled onto something that has eluded others much smarter than me. The path seems obvious in hindsight, but was far from obvious at that time. To keep moving down this road meant risking the alienation of my doctors, the team that had done so much for me over the years — especially Dr. Internal who had saved my life in 1999 and done so much more over the years. To continue this way would be to challenge his education, experience and expertise. Given all I had to deal with, not waking up each day knowing that you have good medical support is frightening.

The support needed came, though, from my kids, my partner and the therapist I had engaged months earlier to help me cope with chronic pain and autonomic neuropathy — long before the breakthrough discovery. Elaine provided critical perspective about how to handle my obvious challenge to the medical community and prevailing "wisdom".

Anyone true to his/her scientific training should not

be offended by a challenge grounded in substance. In fact, she added, the best will rise to the occasion, grasp onto the little kernel of possibility and ride it as far as possible.

By the time Elaine coached me forward, I had already started weaning myself off many medications, with the knowledge of Dr. Internal. He was very supportive of my goal of getting off as many medications as possible, even if the foundation for my effort was simply wacky. We both agreed that even if the entire "link" was one of self-delusion, so what? If some mind games allowed me to function pain-free and drug-free, who cares?

An interesting side issue emerged at this point. People I had known for years and who had seen me suffer so, started making comments about how good I looked: relaxed, refreshed and younger. Each compliment, though, came with the same question, What are you doing? Are you taking something new? I shied away from ever answering the question. It would have brought up too many other questions and most people would have again questioned my sanity. So I kept quiet and continued to use myself as a test subject for my own treatment.

By mid March, I had weaned off the pain medications, had a 10-week history of no pain or attacks, and a far-more detailed set of questions and analysis to present to my doctors. Dr. Internal's response was frustrating, though understandable. I believe, he said, that it works for you. And, I can see how you arrive logically at each point in your argument. It does make some sense, though it goes against just about everything I know from practice. Do what you want, but I am a doctor, not a researcher, and I have no ability to pursue this with or for you.

Well, damn. My endocrinologist, however, surprised me by taking the opposite tack. He called me into his office, I thought, to check up on my thyroid medication so I could renew the prescription for the hormone replacement. Instead, he focused entirely on my report and hypothesis. After talking about it for some time, he started digging through research papers, notes, articles and books looking for some links, a clue here or there to help him understand it better.

I believe you, he said. It defies conventional wisdom, but I really believe you are on to something. I just don't know where to go next, but I am going to help you get there. I am very, very curious about this.

Frustrated with not being able to find anything in his immediate grasp to latch onto, he sat back and started thumbing through his Rolodex. A few minutes later, he started punching numbers in his phone, talking briefly to a few people in an effort to establish some contacts. Then a smile crossed his face and he intoned, "I am going to take this to the National Institutes of Health. I have a connection to a lead researcher there and I am going to take this to them."

Wow. I couldn't have been any happier. Well, not until a few weeks later when he called me early on a Sunday morning after a returning from the Middle East less than 12 hours earlier.

"I've got some good news and some bad news," he offered. The good news? "You're not crazy." Thanks. His contact essentially confirmed the validity of my argument by noting that the NIH had known for a few years of the possible link of unexpectedly high low glucose levels linked to autonomic neuropathy. "This was the first he knew of someone with evidence of these problems in the 90+ range, but it is quite possible." The evidence, my doctor understood, pointed to an abnormal reaction between insulin levels and adrenaline.

The bad news? Due to budget cuts and constraints imposed by current events, the NIH could not pursue this matter further and could not even consider seeing me as a patient or test subject. The advice from the NIH researcher? Tell your patient to keep going and tell others about his experiences.

Obviously, I heeded that advice and you are holding in your hands the culmination of my efforts to date.

At that one moment in my journey, on that Sunday morning, so many thoughts crowded into my mind. Why me?

dominates our thoughts when the news is bad. But this was indeed great news. So, why me? What made my situation so different, so unique as to warrant the possibility of stumbling onto a major discovery that could improve the lives of thousands — maybe millions — of people? I am not a doctor. I am not a research scientist. How could I have accomplished this task?

These thoughts played out against memories, painful memories, of the cardiac arrest in 1999 and the years of misery that followed. Day after day, night followed by night I suffered with pain and a host of malfunctioning body parts. I certainly never thought that it was fair for me to have to have suffered through all of that. Perhaps, I pondered, a divine balancing act is underway. To accept the gift, you have to accept the suffering.

Why had I not succumbed spiritually, emotionally, mentally to the pain and misery — let alone physically? The simple answer: I didn't want to. My wonderful family didn't want me to. My doctors didn't want me to even if they held out no real answers nor effective treatment.

I find the overuse of the word "empowerment" annoying and bordering on trite. In this case, though, it works. Those closest to me asked "only" that I fight the illness and suffering. Just smile through the pain. My parents provided me with an excellent education both at home and in the classroom. My experiences built on that foundation. Somewhere, somehow, the right doors had opened while others had closed. Paths taken while others not followed. It all lead to the moment I now experienced on a sunny, warm Sunday morning.

Ask not why. Simply proceed.

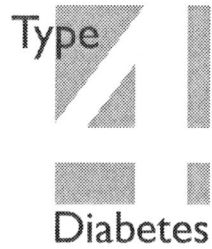

Type 4 Diabetes

Chapter 11

- High & Low Glucose

- Excess Insulin

- Elevated Adrenaline

- Defining Type 4 Diabetes

Chapter 11
Conclusion ... To Date

My journey took me a long way: from the brief glimpse of the after-life through years of pain and misery to a point of discovery and breakthrough. Indeed, I had come a long way. But, the journey is just beginning.

I am not a doctor. I am a patient. And, I have a story to tell. Many may not want to hear it. Many may dismiss it. But, others will benefit. Others will be spared. You can't ask for more than that in one life.

My efforts, my inspiration, my struggle, my pain, and my anxiety were vindicated, rewarded and validated. My frustration? Not being able to tell the world all at once. My mission? To do whatever I can to stoke the intellectual fires within the health care community, to ignite and unite people with autonomic neuropathy, diabetes and low blood sugar, their caregivers and anyone who suspects he or she might be burdened with these problems to demand that their interests be considered.

Type 4 Diabetes = the high glucose complications of diabetes + the low glucose complications of hypoglycemia + the complications of autonomic neuropathy

THE HIGH GLUCOSE COMPLICATIONS

The dangers of high glucose need little elaboration. Over time improperly managed high levels of blood sugar kills. It destroys kidneys, robs people of their vision, leads to amputations and promotes cardiovascular disease. Every adult should know his/her fasting glucose level. Make sure the test is performed at least once a year at the time of your annual physical. Not planning to see your doctor soon? Buy a test kit now. If your fasting level is 100 or more SEE YOUR DOCTOR!

THE LOW GLUCOSE COMPLICATIONS

Though the dangers of high blood sugar levels are well documented and publicized, the risks develop over time – except in cases of extreme high levels. The opposite is true with low levels: the spectrum of dangers is not well understood, but the dangers tend to be more immediate.

- Shakiness, anxiety, nervousness, tremor

- Palpitations and other heart arrhythmias

- Sweating, feeling of warmth or coldness, clamminess

- Dilated pupils

- Hunger or nausea, vomiting, abdominal discomfort

- Impaired judgment

- Personality change, anxiety, moodiness, depression, crying, fear of dying

- Negativism, irritability, belligerence, combativeness, rage

- Fatigue, weakness, apathy, lethargy, daydreaming, sleep

- Confusion, amnesia, dizziness, delirium

- Staring, "glassy" look, blurred vision, double vision

- Difficulty speaking, slurred speech, lack of coordination, sometimes mistaken for "drunkenness"

- Seizures, stupor, coma

THE COMPLICATIONS OF AUTONOMIC NEUROPATHY

- Urinary bladder

- Bladder incontinence or urine retention

- Gastrointestinal tract

- Difficulty in swallowing

- Abdominal pain

- Nausea

- Vomiting

- Fecal incontinence

- Gastroparesis (too long to digest food)

- Improper absorption of nutrient in the intestines

- Diarrhea

- Constipation

- Cardiovascular system

- Disturbances of heart rate (tachycardia and/or bradycardia)

- Orthostatic hypotension (problem with standing)

- Inadequate increase of heart rate on exertion

- Other

- Erectile impotence

- Hypoglycemia unawareness

LOW GLUCOSE + AUTONOMIC NEUROPATHY COMPLICATIONS

I have experienced every complication and symptom listed above for both low glucose and autonomic neuropathy. Mere coincidence? I don't believe so. As already noted, there has been a sharp increase in the number of diabetes patients diagnosed with autonomic neuropathy in the last two decades. Studies now show that more than 60% of patients with diabetes have or can expect to develop symptoms of autonomic neuropathy.

Why the increase? Is it due to better diagnostic techniques and understanding of autonomic neuropathy? Yes, that can be one answer. But, I suspect something else is in play. The same 20+ years of increase in autonomic neuropathy also corresponds with the time frame during which "designer" insulin therapies and a wide spectrum of oral Type 2 medications have come available.

Prior to 1982, the only insulin available to doctors in treating diabetes came from animals (cow, horse, pig and fish). Though widely effective, animal-based insulin does produce allergic reactions in some people and limits treatment options. The introduction of DNA-engineered insulin, Humulin, by Eli Lilly in 1982, opened the door to an array of different types of insulin: quick-acting, short-acting, intermediate-acting, long-acting and various combinations. Armed with this array, doctors have the ability to prescribe a very specific regime of insulin therapy for each patient aimed at successfully lowering glucose levels to or even below levels found in people without diabetes.

Since the 1950s, doctors have been able to prescribe an oral medication to help stimulate the beta cells in the pancreas to produce more insulin. Known as Sulfonylureas, these drugs stood alone until the 1980s when four new classes of medications began to emerge. These drugs treat Type 2 Diabetes through stimulation of the beta cells to increase insulin, depressing the action of the liver in releasing glucose, improving the cellular absorption of glucose, slowing the breakdown of starches or a combination of several approaches.

Given the new insulin therapies and oral medications, responsible medical practice dictated that doctors aggressively use these tools to drive every possible patient away from the risks of high glucose levels – as far away as possible.

Perhaps the aggressive treatment went too far.

PUTTING IT ALL TOGETHER

1. In 1999, I experienced a cardiac arrest and the implanting of a pacemaker. The diagnosis was autonomic neuropathy.

2. In the first three years that followed, I suffered through every symptom of autonomic neuropathy. There were no effective treatments, only approaches to managing the worst of the pain with large doses of Neurontin and other medications. At best these drugs only worked 50% of the time, reducing most, but not all of the pain and other symptoms.

3. In 2004 I began to treat the problems of autonomic neuropathy more effectively, not with medications, but through lifestyle changes: more sleep, more exercise and tighter control over my diet. These are the same essential steps a patient with prediabetes should take to delay or prevent the onset of Type 2, and many if not most patients with Type 2 can do so rather than take drugs.

4. In 2005, the first warning signs of diabetes appeared. I began to test my blood sugar daily.

5. In the fall of 2005, I discovered that the worst symptoms of autonomic neuropa-

thy correlated with lower than my normal glucose levels.

6. Just before New Year's 2005 I discovered that I could completely manage the autonomic neuropathy symptoms by elevating my base glucose levels to 100.

7. At first, my routine consisted of testing up to eight times each day

8. If the meter reading was below 100, I dissolved 4 grams of quick dissolving glucose tablets on my tongue, waited 15 minutes and tested again.

9. If the meter reading was below 90, I dissolved 8 grams; below 80, 12 grams.

10. Within six months, I could well predict the meter reading based on how I felt. Many times now, I just skip the reading and go for the glucose.

11. In the months that followed, my glucose "highs" dropped from 300 to the mid-100s.

12. I learned in April 2006 that at least one researcher at NIH knew of a link between insulin and adrenalin that could explain most if not all of these circumstances.

13. In 2006, I withdrew from all of my medications successfully without any recurrence

of the 24/7 pain and complications of autonomic neuropathy.

Yes, there still are limits past which my body does not want to go. If I do not get enough sleep over a period of days, if I push myself too hard physically, if I spend too much time working and coding websites, I will suffer. Headaches will start again and I will feel some pain in my legs. But, I am not in my 20s anymore.

When I push too hard the key warning sign, though, is that I will experience problems in elevating my base (basal) glucose level to 100 and maintaining it in that range. But, my routine outlined in the steps above works. I just have to be patient and follow the procedure several times a day after a prolonged period of pushing myself.

ONE POSSIBLE THEORY

"Your problem involves an aberrant insulin-adrenaline reaction." When I first heard the phrase from my endocrinologist, repeating what he had heard from the NIH, it sounded reasonable. Why not? Insulin and adrenaline are key hormones that must work properly to keep our bodies in balance. I knew that much. How specifically, though, did one work with the other — or in my case not work with each other — to cause neuropathic pain and complications?

For months that followed I searched extensively for information that would shed some light on the theory. One day, after hours of deep Web-based research, I came across the writings of Dr. R. Paul St. Amand. With 50 years teaching experience at in the Department of Endocrinology at Los Angeles Harbor/UCLA, Dr. Amand is widely known for his expertise in fibromyalgia. Recognized in 1987 by the American Medical Association, fibromyalgia is a debilitating chronic syndrome characterized by diffuse or specific muscle, joint, or bone pain, fatigue, and a wide range of other symptoms.

Perhaps coincidentally many of symptoms of fibromyalgia mirror those of hypoglycemia. In his years of study, Dr. St. Amand noted a strong correlation between the two diseases or syndromes. His efforts to help patients has led the doctor into detailed analyses of hypoglycemia and, in doing so, to suggest a theory to explain how I could treat my autonomic neuropathy symptoms with just glucose — and maybe how many of those suffering from fibromyalgia could discover some relief.

> There are two ways to produce low blood sugar. The most obvious way is by an excess of insulin, but it an also be caused by delayed or inadequate hormonal responses that are supposed to put a brake on rapidly falling sugar. The latter are known as counter-regulatory hormones because they normally stop the over exuberant attacks of insulin. All kids of freakish possibilities exist, because a little too much of this or too little of that creates a whole spectrum of stresses. Combinations of various defects viciously strain a variety of cells.

> There are four important counter-regulatory hormones, but adrenaline (epinephrine) is the ultimate weapon, and the final safety net. If either insulin or adrenaline is released in delayed, inadequate, or excessive amounts, the other one must decrease or increase its output to avoid hypoglycemia. They dance together, but at opposite ends of the ballroom. It is this bad choreography that causes the distinctive symptoms in susceptible people.[1]

Insulin drives blood sugar down by opening doors to cells to absorb glucose. Adrenalin pushes it back up. It's a natural balancing act that takes place every second in a healthy body. In reactive people, a trigger event occurs leading to a higher-than-normal release of insulin into the system. Blood sugar starts falling rapidly. The brain reacts "out of fear" of being deprived of critical "energy" and stimulates the release of counter-regulatory hormones: growth hormone, glucagon and cortisol. However, since these hormones cannot respond fast enough, a "super-charged" release of adrenaline is stimulated stopping the fall of blood sugar within one to two minutes.

Adrenaline, sometimes known as the "fight-or-flight" hormone, "punishes" the body in an unnecessarily large release by creating heart pounding, sweating, acute anxiety, shaking tremors and pressure headaches.

Following on what Dr. St. Amand writes, I can understand how raising my glucose level could halt my symptoms of autonomic neuropathy. The rapid-acting glucose tablet quickly puts enough sugar into my system to prevent inappropriately large releases of adrenaline. No longer fearing energy starvation, the brain "backs down."

Without the braking intervention of oral glucose, my reactive system would continue on a roller-coaster cycle of errant insulin and adrenaline releases. After a period of time, this cycle must wear on the organs of the body. The result? Pain and organ malfunctions. Perhaps what I experienced in 1999 and the years that followed was a series of acute episodes of errant insulin-adrenalin reactions.

In that, I can't be alone. There must be many, many others who experience the same. Our carb-loaded diets set the stage for stressing the intricately balanced glucose metabolism process. Our over zealous response in driving our glucose levels as low as possible raises the curtain. Too much sugar. Too little sugar. Just maybe it is a recipe for trouble.

As Sherlock Holmes Would Say ...

In my mind, no doubt exists about what this all means. Naturally, other people may be skeptics. To those I say, look at the possible choices:

1. I was misdiagnosed in 1999 and didn't have autonomic neuropathy. But, then why the pacemaker and why did I present with the entire range of autonomic neuropathy symptoms? No, autonomic neuropathy was the correct diagnosis – at least as it was understood.

2. My doctors have been treating me for the wrong disease, or incorrectly for the appropriate disease, since 1999. No. These are educated, competent, highly regarded medical specialists. None of them would knowingly allow me to suffer persistent high levels of pain when a simple treatment would have ended the pain. And, my treatment was the result of multiple doctors examining me 6-12 times a year and sharing the results with each other.

3. All the pain and subsequent relief is imagined. OK. That might be possible. But, then we're faced with the reality that I am not a unique individual in my symptoms. If I can get my pain to go away with "mental tricks" then a lot of people could benefit from psychotherapy to treat autonomic neuropathy.

In the persona of Sherlock Holmes, Arthur Conan Doyle wrote: "when you have eliminated the impossible, whatever remains, however improbable, must be the truth."

Therefore,

4. I have stumbled onto a new understanding of glucose metabolism and the problems that result from levels that are low, although much higher than previously considered as the range within which one experiences complications of hypoglycemia. These complications previously have been labeled as symptoms of autonomic neuropathy. (Though, in the absence of faulty glucose metabolism, these problems may still be presented and considered as autonomic neuropathy.)

Given that, I offer for consideration a redefinition of diabetes as a disease of glucose metabolism with inherent, serious complications as a result of both higher than normal and lower than normal levels of glucose in the blood. For the moment, let's call the low-end complications Type 4 Diabetes.

Let the formal research begin. Please.

Type 4 Diabetes. Elevated insulin levels leading to low blood sugar, chronic pain and related complications of the nervous system.

In Addition

▓ Endnotes

1. Paul St. Amand, <u>What Your Doctor May Not Tell You About Fibromyalgia</u> (New York: Warner, 2006) p. 105

> You can locate updated information
> and additional links by visiting:
> www.type4diabetes.com.

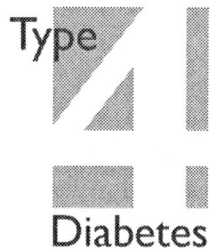

Postscript

Postscript

On September 28, 2006, a smiling medical technician held a sensor device over my chest as she uploaded the information from my Medtronic pacemaker to the computer on the stand to my right. Fourteen months had elapsed since the last pacemaker check — just 434 days, but a 2nd lifetime ago.

Why, she asked, did I have a pacemaker? If I needed one in the years past, what had changed? Why was my pacemaker basically only "turning on" at night when my natural pulse was dropping below the 60 beats per minute? — the threshold point at which the pacemaker kicks in. What had changed so much inside of me?

In the initial years that followed October 15, 1999, my pacemaker took over the task of providing a steady nerve impulse to my heart 70% of the time. On average over the last 14 months, it swung into action less than 30% of time. Looking ahead, the profile suggested 10% or less usage.

To those who doubt the words in this book, and the conclusions I draw, I offer a fundamental challenge: please give me another explanation.

Did I coerce my doctors into implanting a pacemaker? Did I conspire with Medtronic or my cardiologists to fake the results of my last pacemaker reading? If it is all in my head, please tell me how one can turn "on" or "off" a heart beat?

Or perhaps I have inadvertently discovered something significant.

I am not a doctor. I am a patient. And I am eager to continue learning.

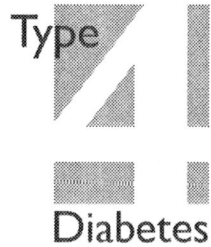

Type
Diabetes

Appendices

Appendix A
CARBS & GLUCOSE.
INSULIN & ADRENALINE.

The glucose link — from the carbohydrates you eat to storage and use in your cells — is well understood. Your digestive system breaks down carbs into glucose which then enters your blood stream. Your blood glucose level goes up. Your pancreas produces insulin, a vital hormone that "opens the door" in cells for glucose to enter and then be used as fuel. Insulin also enables glucose to be stored for future use in the liver and fat cells.

Without sufficient insulin, as in Type 1 Diabetes, your body cannot absorb glucose produced from carbs for use as fuel. In Type 2, you may have both insufficient amounts of insulin as well as the cellular "doors" for glucose not "opening" properly (insulin resistance).

When you have excessive amounts of insulin in your system, your blood glucose level drop too low. Too much glucose is being stored and not enough remains freely available for use as immediate energy.

Adrenaline, along with several other hormones, serves as a "brake" on falling glucose levels by limiting the action of insulin. Balanced together, these hormones keep your system functioning properly.

In Type 4, excessive insulin lowers glucose levels too low and too quickly and results in excessive adrenaline being produced. In some people, excessive adrenaline causes severe side effects and initiates a roller coaster ride of high/low levels of insulin and adrenaline along with alternating periods of hyperglycemia (too much blood sugar) and hypoglycemia (too little).

The Type 4 Diabetes Link

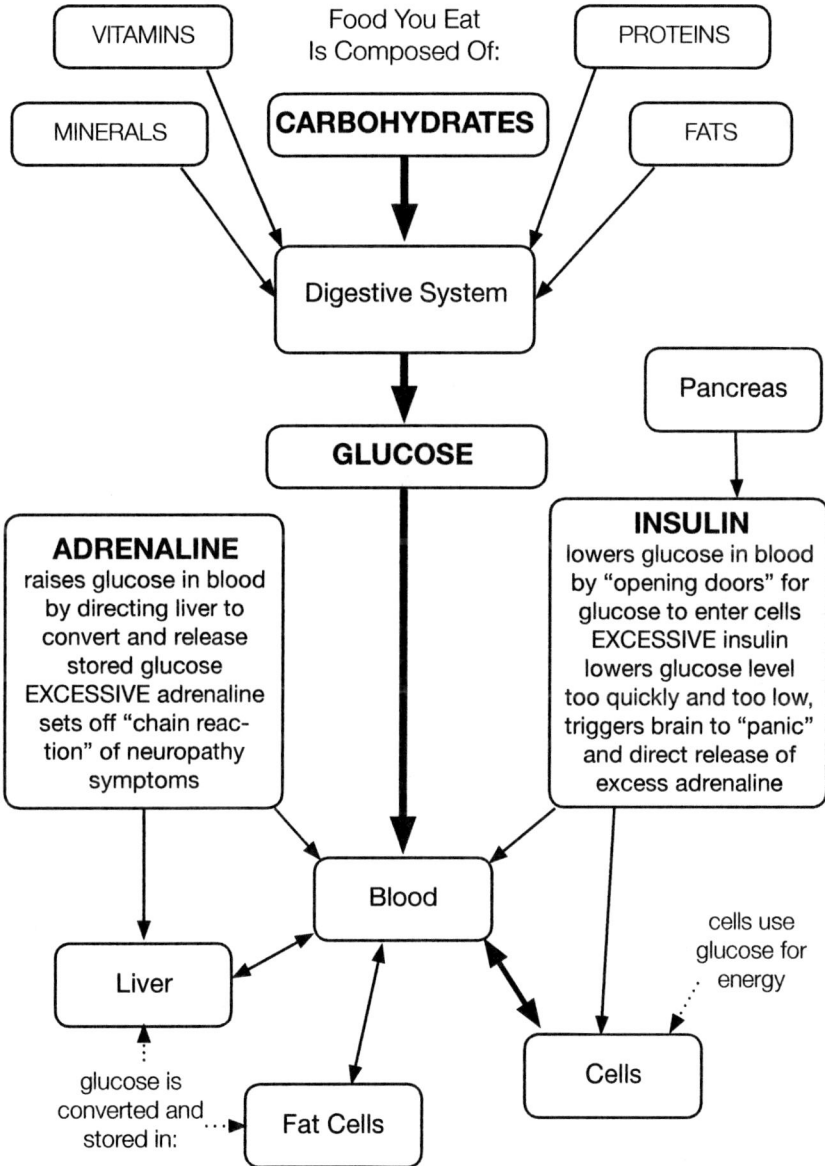

VITAMINS

Food You Eat
Is Composed Of:

PROTEINS

MINERALS

CARBOHYDRATES

FATS

Digestive System

Pancreas

GLUCOSE

INSULIN
lowers glucose in blood
by "opening doors" for
glucose to enter cells
EXCESSIVE insulin
lowers glucose level
too quickly and too low,
triggers brain to "panic"
and direct release of
excess adrenaline

ADRENALINE
raises glucose in blood
by directing liver to
convert and release
stored glucose
EXCESSIVE adrenaline
sets off "chain reac-
tion" of neuropathy
symptoms

Blood

cells use
glucose for
energy

Liver

Cells

glucose is
converted and
stored in:

Fat Cells

Appendix B
TYPE 4 DIABETES DIAGNOSIS
AND MANAGEMENT PLAN

Being at the forefront in the understanding and management of Type 4 presents a special challenge. Whereas with most serious diseases you can rely on the experience of countless others to guide the decision-making and treatment plan, no such direct resource exists here — with the sole exception of this author.

Instead, a foundation of knowledge can built on the experiences of people who have successfully dealt with diabetes, neuropathy and the symptoms of hypoglycemia. In presenting this plan, I have combined this knowledge with my own experiences over the last seven years.

As I have stated repeatedly throughout this book, I assuredly am not alone in confronting this combination of symptoms, syndromes and diseases. By linking this book to an open community blog/website I sincerely hope and fully expect that hundreds, perhaps thousands, will soon share their experiences, ideas and suggestions for mutual benefit. You are invited to visit the site, gain as much as you can from the posted content and contribute, if you so wish, to the growing book of knowledge.

www.Type4Diabetes.com

7 STEPS TO DIAGNOSIS AND MANAGEMENT

1. Learning

2. Testing

3. Tracking

4. Transferring

5. Dieting

6. Exercising

7. Treating

DIAGNOSIS: FOCUS ON STEPS 1-3

Do I have symptoms of diabetes, neuropathy and/or hypoglycemia? Are these symptoms distinct or related? Could my symptoms be interrelated and fall into the category of Type 4 diabetes — and possibly be treated successfully with small amounts of glucose?

Theses and many more questions should be of paramount importance to you if you have taken the time to read this book. While the questions are obvious, the answers, at this point, are not very clear.

As noted throughout this book, I cannot be — most certainly I am not — unique in having overlapping symptoms of diabetes, neuropathy and hypoglycemia. The physicians that have worked with me now believe that there are thousands, perhaps millions, of others who share the same problems and can be treated in the same way.

Where do you begin?

1. **Learning**. If you suspect that you may be suffering from Type 4, or are a caregiver for someone who could be, the first step is, indeed, knowledge:

   a. Read this book and visit the website.

   b. Follow the links in this book to content-rich sites focusing on diabetes, neuropathy, hypoglycemia and even Alzheimer's and fibromyalgia.

   c. Visit bookstores (online and physical) that abound in reference materials on these subjects.

   d. Check out your local library.

   e. Go see your physician.

2. **Testing**. If you don't have a home glucose meter, go buy one now. Chapter 7 provides insights into meters as well as links to sites and stores where you can easily purchase a meter that meets your needs and budget.

3. **Tracking**. As discussed in Chapter 7, go simple (pencil and paper) or go geek (computer program) as long as you track all relevant information.

   a. In the following appendix, you will find a paper-based tracking log offering a convenient method for keeping tabs of your glucose readings as well as symptoms of neuropathy and low blood sugar plus exercise, diet and additional comments. Had I been tracking my diabetes test results and neuropathy medications/symptoms on a combined log such as this, most certainly I would realized the relationship between the two diseases much sooner.

b. Track your results and fill in the key information for at least four weeks.

c. Start tracking how many calories and carbs you consume at each meal. A good beginning assist is the *Complete Guide to Carb Counting* from the American Diabetes Association.

d. Make special notes about your caffeine and alcohol consumption. Really. As with many others, I consider a good day to be built around a great cup of coffee in the morning, a large glass of iced tea at lunch and a nice wine at dinner. However, caffeine and alcohol should be considered potent drugs that can quickly and adversely impact your blood glucose level as well as bring on symptoms of neuropathy and/or hypoglycemia in certain people. In my case, both alcohol and caffeine can lower my glucose levels too quickly and bring on headaches and other symptoms. I have to limit and balance my consumption of each.

e. Begin to look for patterns and oddities.

  - How do you feel when your glucose levels are low?

  - How do you feel when your levels are high?

  - How do you feel in the morning and what are your glucose levels?

  - Does your glucose level go up two hours after breakfast?

  - What happens to your post-breakfast levels when you change your morning diet?

  - When do you get a headache, what is your glucose level?

  - Do you have other symptoms when you have a headache?

- Can you begin to predict glucose levels based on other symptoms and factors such as diet and exercise?

MANAGEMENT: FOCUS ON STEPS 4-7

About testing and tracking: We all ask the same questions in time: Do I need to track all of this several time each day? Can I just test and track once a day? When can I skip a day or so?

- In the beginning, the answer is simple: Yes, you need to test your glucose and track your wellness index several times each and every day, and track your exercises and diet daily. You need this information and if you don't write it down immediately, you are bound to forget important information.
- How long have I been tracking in this much detail? As of this printing, for more than a year. Do I occasionally miss a glucose test or observation? Of course and I don't worry about it. Even though I can predict with great accuracy my glucose test results based on how I feel and the extent to which I have experienced and my recent diet, I still want to know more. Knowledge is indeed power.

4. **Transferring**. As of this printing, I only know of a handful of physicians who concur with the focus of this book. Undoubtedly, your physician or health care provider is going to be skeptical. Hopefully he or she will at least be intrigued and willing to seriously consider your informed concerns and requests for assistance. Regardless of how deep the initial skepticism may be, you should never attempt to self-diagnose or treat the symptoms covered in Type 4 Diabetes on your own. There are many diseases with similar symptoms that require immediate medical attention and only a trained physician can perform the necessary tests to ascertain your

exact medical issues. As I have noted several times, I indeed followed my own path in treating my illnesses. But, I always kept at least one of my doctors informed as to what I was doing and what was occurring. I visited a doctor each month and necessary blood and other tests were performed to monitor my progress.

5. **Dieting**. It is worth repeating over and over again. Fact: most patients with Type 2 diabetes can maintain good blood glucose levels without insulin and oral medications. And, most people with prediabetes can delay or even prevent the onset of Type 2 without drugs. Diet and exercise are the keys.

   a. Get a check up and ask your doctor for your ideal weight and her or his recommendations on reaching that weight.

   b. Enlist the services of a dietician or nutritionist either on your own or through a local diabetes or heart support group or medical center.

   c. Discover new recipes for healthy diabetes and heart eating. A good beginning point is *The Diabetes & Heart Healthy Cookbook* published jointly by the American Diabetes Association and the American Heart Association.

   d. Through tracking, I have discovered that a diet consisting of of about 65 grams of carbs for breakfast works best for me:
      - Cranberry juice   (33 grams of carbs)
      - Whole grain granola   (22 grams of carbs)
      - Sugar-free and fat-free yogurt   (10 grams of carbs)
      Some dieticians might take exception to a breakfast with this many carbs. But, I have made it a weekday routine, I digest it well, it is heart-healthy and my glucose levels respond predictably – it drops. So I eat a small mid-morning snack to push my glucose levels back up.

Nighttime Note: I also have added a bedtime snack, something very new for me. But, I only do so when my glucose level is below 100 at bedtime or I have exercised in the evening. The snack is a glucose-stabilizing bar such as ExtendBar (www.extendbar.com). These bars take up to nine hours to digest so that glucose is released over time into your system.

6. **Exercising.** I believe that many people who avoid consistent exercise may have some form of neuropathy or even Type 4 Diabetes. I have always believed in the importance of exercise since my youth, but just couldn't understand nor manage the frequent downsides of exercise. I remember at one point in my life complaining to a doctor that the day after a strenuous workout always felt as if I was coming down with a bad cold or the flu. I believe his words were more or less "You're nuts."

   a. The need for all adults to exercise is without question – and it is not that difficult to achieve the minimum exercise requirements set forth by experts in diabetes and cardiovascular health. A 30-minute walk, 3-5 days a week is a great beginning.

7. **Treating.** Any type of diabetes is a serious, life-long disease. There is no cure for diabetes. The steps outlined above can go a long way to managing Type 4 Diabetes as well as Type 2. But, you may require the addition of specific medications, insulin or, in the case of Type 4, glucose.

   a. Type 4 and Glucose. Based on my own testing and tracking, I learned that symptoms of neuropathy and hypoglycemia begin when my glucose drops rapidly to a level below 100. The higher my level when the decline begins and the speed at which the glucose declines increases the potential and severity of the pain and complications.

b. When I feel symptoms beginning or note my glucose level falling below 100, I begin to treat the Type 4 with 4 -8 milligrams of quick-dissolving glucose. (These tablets are available from most pharmacies or supermarkets, as well as online merchants such as drugstore.com.)

c. In most cases, 8 milligrams is enough to break the cycle and prevent the onset of complications. Before reading St. Amand's work on errant insulin-glucose reactions, I accepted, but did not understand how so little glucose could prevent any further symptoms and complications. Based on his theory, it makes sense that one to two work by "tricking the brain" into realizing that there still is sufficient glucose available to keep functioning.

d. Until further evidence is available through research or shared experiences, we don't know if my threshold level is high, low or about the same for most people who have Type 4. *Please help in this process* by sharing your experiences, testing and tracking with others via the blog/website: www.type4diabetes.com.

Appendix C
TYPE 4 DIABETES 30-DAY TRACKING LOG

Using the Daily Tracking Log only takes a few minutes each day, but the rewards can be significant. Set a target number of days for your tracking; I recommend one month. Keep the log in a convenient place with your glucose meter.

1. **Date**: enter today's date and circle the day of the week.
2. **Meter Readings**: The three key times are Fasting (before breakfast, after not eating for eat least eight hours), Post-breakfast (2 or so hours after finishing breakfast) and Bedtime (just before going to sleep). You can track at other times around meals and exercise as needed.
3. **Wellness Index**: How do you feel at these times? **M**: miserable, **S-S**: so-so, **G**: good, **VG**: very good.
4. **Symptoms**: **Pain**, **LH**: lightheaded, **Dg**: indigestion or other gastrointestinal problems, **Co**: cognitive, are you having problems thinking?
5. **Meals**: What did you eat? Key things to track are total amount of carbs and calories for each mean and snack. Nighttime: did you eat a glucose-stabilizing snack such as ExtendBar?
6. **Exercise**: what **Time** of the day did you exercise? The **Type** (walking, yoga, swimming, weights and how strenuous), **Duration** (how much time spent) and **Comments** (easy, hard today).
7. **Notes**: additional space for tracking items above as well as general comments about how you felt during the day, changes that took place.

Type 4 Diabetes Daily Tracking Log

Date		S M T W Th F S		
Meter Readings		**Wellness Index**	**Pain LH Dg Co**	**Meals**
Fasting Glucose		M S-S G VG		Breakfast
Post-breakfast		M S-S G VG		Snack
Other daytime		M S-S G VG		Lunch
Other daytime		M S-S G VG		Dinner
Other daytime		M S-S G VG		Snack
Bedtime		M S-S G VG		Nighttime

Exercise	**Time**	**Type**		**Duration**	**Comments**

Notes

Type 4 Diabetes Daily Tracking Log

Date		S M T W Th F S		
Meter Readings		**Wellness Index**	**Pain LH Dg Co**	**Meals**
Fasting Glucose		M S-S G VG		Breakfast
Post-breakfast		M S-S G VG		Snack
Other daytime		M S-S G VG		Lunch
Other daytime		M S-S G VG		Dinner
Other daytime		M S-S G VG		Snack
Bedtime		M S-S G VG		Nighttime

Exercise	**Time**	**Type**		**Duration**	**Comments**

Notes

Type 4 Diabetes Daily Tracking Log

Date		S M T W Th F S		
Meter Readings		**Wellness Index**	**Pain LH Dg Co**	**Meals**
Fasting Glucose		M S-S G VG		Breakfast
Post-breakfast		M S-S G VG		Snack
Other daytime		M S-S G VG		Lunch
Other daytime		M S-S G VG		Dinner
Other daytime		M S-S G VG		Snack
Bedtime		M S-S G VG		Nighttime

Exercise	**Time**	**Type**		**Duration**	**Comments**

Notes

Type 4 Diabetes Daily Tracking Log

Date		S M T W Th F S		
Meter Readings		**Wellness Index**	**Pain LH Dg Co**	**Meals**	
Fasting Glucose		M S-S G VG		Breakfast	
Post-breakfast		M S-S G VG		Snack	
Other daytime		M S-S G VG		Lunch	
Other daytime		M S-S G VG		Dinner	
Other daytime		M S-S G VG		Snack	
Bedtime		M S-S G VG		Nighttime	

Exercise	**Time**	**Type**		**Duration**	**Comments**

Notes

Type 4 Diabetes Daily Tracking Log

Date		S M T W Th F S		
Meter Readings		**Wellness Index**	**Pain LH Dg Co**	**Meals**	
Fasting Glucose		M S-S G VG		Breakfast	
Post-breakfast		M S-S G VG		Snack	
Other daytime		M S-S G VG		Lunch	
Other daytime		M S-S G VG		Dinner	
Other daytime		M S-S G VG		Snack	
Bedtime		M S-S G VG		Nighttime	

Exercise	**Time**	**Type**		**Duration**	**Comments**

Notes

Type 4 Diabetes Daily Tracking Log

Date		S M T W Th F S		
Meter Readings		**Wellness Index**	**Pain LH Dg Co**	**Meals**	
Fasting Glucose		M S-S G VG		Breakfast	
Post-breakfast		M S-S G VG		Snack	
Other daytime		M S-S G VG		Lunch	
Other daytime		M S-S G VG		Dinner	
Other daytime		M S-S G VG		Snack	
Bedtime		M S-S G VG		Nighttime	

Exercise	**Time**	**Type**		**Duration**	**Comments**

Notes

Type 4 Diabetes Daily Tracking Log

Date		S M T W Th F S			
Meter Readings		**Wellness Index**	**Pain LH Dg Co**	**Meals**	
Fasting Glucose		M S-S G VG		Breakfast	
Post-breakfast		M S-S G VG		Snack	
Other daytime		M S-S G VG		Lunch	
Other daytime		M S-S G VG		Dinner	
Other daytime		M S-S G VG		Snack	
Bedtime		M S-S G VG		Nighttime	

Exercise	Time	Type		Duration	Comments

Notes

Type 4 Diabetes Daily Tracking Log

Date		S M T W Th F S			
Meter Readings		**Wellness Index**	**Pain LH Dg Co**	**Meals**	
Fasting Glucose		M S-S G VG		Breakfast	
Post-breakfast		M S-S G VG		Snack	
Other daytime		M S-S G VG		Lunch	
Other daytime		M S-S G VG		Dinner	
Other daytime		M S-S G VG		Snack	
Bedtime		M S-S G VG		Nighttime	

Exercise	Time	Type		Duration	Comments

Notes

Type 4 Diabetes Daily Tracking Log

Date		S M T W Th F S			
Meter Readings		**Wellness Index**	**Pain LH Dg Co**	**Meals**	
Fasting Glucose		M S-S G VG		Breakfast	
Post-breakfast		M S-S G VG		Snack	
Other daytime		M S-S G VG		Lunch	
Other daytime		M S-S G VG		Dinner	
Other daytime		M S-S G VG		Snack	
Bedtime		M S-S G VG		Nighttime	

Exercise	Time	Type		Duration	Comments

Notes

Type 4 Diabetes Daily Tracking Log

Date		S M T W Th F S			
Meter Readings		**Wellness Index**	**Pain LH Dg Co**	**Meals**	
Fasting Glucose		M S-S G VG		Breakfast	
Post-breakfast		M S-S G VG		Snack	
Other daytime		M S-S G VG		Lunch	
Other daytime		M S-S G VG		Dinner	
Other daytime		M S-S G VG		Snack	
Bedtime		M S-S G VG		Nighttime	

Exercise	**Time**	**Type**		**Duration**	**Comments**

Notes

Type 4 Diabetes Daily Tracking Log

Date		S M T W Th F S			
Meter Readings		**Wellness Index**	**Pain LH Dg Co**	**Meals**	
Fasting Glucose		M S-S G VG		Breakfast	
Post-breakfast		M S-S G VG		Snack	
Other daytime		M S-S G VG		Lunch	
Other daytime		M S-S G VG		Dinner	
Other daytime		M S-S G VG		Snack	
Bedtime		M S-S G VG		Nighttime	

Exercise	**Time**	**Type**		**Duration**	**Comments**

Notes

Type 4 Diabetes Daily Tracking Log

Date		S M T W Th F S			
Meter Readings		**Wellness Index**	**Pain LH Dg Co**	**Meals**	
Fasting Glucose		M S-S G VG		Breakfast	
Post-breakfast		M S-S G VG		Snack	
Other daytime		M S-S G VG		Lunch	
Other daytime		M S-S G VG		Dinner	
Other daytime		M S-S G VG		Snack	
Bedtime		M S-S G VG		Nighttime	

Exercise	**Time**	**Type**		**Duration**	**Comments**

Notes

Type 4 Diabetes Daily Tracking Log

Date		S M T W Th F S		
Meter Readings		**Wellness Index**	**Pain LH Dg Co**	**Meals**
Fasting Glucose		M S-S G VG		Breakfast
Post-breakfast		M S-S G VG		Snack
Other daytime		M S-S G VG		Lunch
Other daytime		M S-S G VG		Dinner
Other daytime		M S-S G VG		Snack
Bedtime		M S-S G VG		Nighttime

Exercise	**Time**	**Type**		**Duration**	**Comments**

Notes

Type 4 Diabetes Daily Tracking Log

Date		S M T W Th F S		
Meter Readings		**Wellness Index**	**Pain LH Dg Co**	**Meals**
Fasting Glucose		M S-S G VG		Breakfast
Post-breakfast		M S-S G VG		Snack
Other daytime		M S-S G VG		Lunch
Other daytime		M S-S G VG		Dinner
Other daytime		M S-S G VG		Snack
Bedtime		M S-S G VG		Nighttime

Exercise	**Time**	**Type**		**Duration**	**Comments**

Notes

Type 4 Diabetes Daily Tracking Log

Date		S M T W Th F S		
Meter Readings		**Wellness Index**	**Pain LH Dg Co**	**Meals**
Fasting Glucose		M S-S G VG		Breakfast
Post-breakfast		M S-S G VG		Snack
Other daytime		M S-S G VG		Lunch
Other daytime		M S-S G VG		Dinner
Other daytime		M S-S G VG		Snack
Bedtime		M S-S G VG		Nighttime

Exercise	**Time**	**Type**		**Duration**	**Comments**

Notes

Type 4 Diabetes Daily Tracking Log

Date		S M T W Th F S		
Meter Readings		**Wellness Index**	**Pain LH Dg Co**	**Meals**
Fasting Glucose		M S-S G VG		Breakfast
Post-breakfast		M S-S G VG		Snack
Other daytime		M S-S G VG		Lunch
Other daytime		M S-S G VG		Dinner
Other daytime		M S-S G VG		Snack
Bedtime		M S-S G VG		Nighttime

Exercise	**Time**	**Type**		**Duration**	**Comments**

Notes

Type 4 Diabetes Daily Tracking Log

Date		S M T W Th F S		
Meter Readings		**Wellness Index**	**Pain LH Dg Co**	**Meals**
Fasting Glucose		M S-S G VG		Breakfast
Post-breakfast		M S-S G VG		Snack
Other daytime		M S-S G VG		Lunch
Other daytime		M S-S G VG		Dinner
Other daytime		M S-S G VG		Snack
Bedtime		M S-S G VG		Nighttime

Exercise	**Time**	**Type**		**Duration**	**Comments**

Notes

Type 4 Diabetes Daily Tracking Log

Date		S M T W Th F S		
Meter Readings		**Wellness Index**	**Pain LH Dg Co**	**Meals**
Fasting Glucose		M S-S G VG		Breakfast
Post-breakfast		M S-S G VG		Snack
Other daytime		M S-S G VG		Lunch
Other daytime		M S-S G VG		Dinner
Other daytime		M S-S G VG		Snack
Bedtime		M S-S G VG		Nighttime

Exercise	**Time**	**Type**		**Duration**	**Comments**

Notes

Type 4 Diabetes Daily Tracking Log

Date		S M T W Th F S		
Meter Readings		**Wellness Index**	**Pain LH Dg Co**	**Meals**
Fasting Glucose		M S-S G VG		Breakfast
Post-breakfast		M S-S G VG		Snack
Other daytime		M S-S G VG		Lunch
Other daytime		M S-S G VG		Dinner
Other daytime		M S-S G VG		Snack
Bedtime		M S-S G VG		Nighttime

Exercise	**Time**	**Type**		**Duration**	**Comments**

Notes

Type 4 Diabetes Daily Tracking Log

Date		S M T W Th F S		
Meter Readings		**Wellness Index**	**Pain LH Dg Co**	**Meals**
Fasting Glucose		M S-S G VG		Breakfast
Post-breakfast		M S-S G VG		Snack
Other daytime		M S-S G VG		Lunch
Other daytime		M S-S G VG		Dinner
Other daytime		M S-S G VG		Snack
Bedtime		M S-S G VG		Nighttime

Exercise	**Time**	**Type**		**Duration**	**Comments**

Notes

Type 4 Diabetes Daily Tracking Log

Date		S M T W Th F S		
Meter Readings		**Wellness Index**	**Pain LH Dg Co**	**Meals**
Fasting Glucose		M S-S G VG		Breakfast
Post-breakfast		M S-S G VG		Snack
Other daytime		M S-S G VG		Lunch
Other daytime		M S-S G VG		Dinner
Other daytime		M S-S G VG		Snack
Bedtime		M S-S G VG		Nighttime

Exercise	**Time**	**Type**		**Duration**	**Comments**

Notes

Type 4 Diabetes Daily Tracking Log

Date		S M T W Th F S		
Meter Readings		**Wellness Index**	**Pain LH Dg Co**	**Meals**
Fasting Glucose		M S-S G VG		Breakfast
Post-breakfast		M S-S G VG		Snack
Other daytime		M S-S G VG		Lunch
Other daytime		M S-S G VG		Dinner
Other daytime		M S-S G VG		Snack
Bedtime		M S-S G VG		Nighttime

Exercise	**Time**	**Type**		**Duration**	**Comments**

Notes

Type 4 Diabetes Daily Tracking Log

Date		S M T W Th F S		
Meter Readings		**Wellness Index**	**Pain LH Dg Co**	**Meals**
Fasting Glucose		M S-S G VG		Breakfast
Post-breakfast		M S-S G VG		Snack
Other daytime		M S-S G VG		Lunch
Other daytime		M S-S G VG		Dinner
Other daytime		M S-S G VG		Snack
Bedtime		M S-S G VG		Nighttime

Exercise	**Time**	**Type**		**Duration**	**Comments**

Notes

Type 4 Diabetes Daily Tracking Log

Date		S M T W Th F S		
Meter Readings		**Wellness Index**	**Pain LH Dg Co**	**Meals**
Fasting Glucose		M S-S G VG		Breakfast
Post-breakfast		M S-S G VG		Snack
Other daytime		M S-S G VG		Lunch
Other daytime		M S-S G VG		Dinner
Other daytime		M S-S G VG		Snack
Bedtime		M S-S G VG		Nighttime

Exercise	**Time**	**Type**		**Duration**	**Comments**

Notes

Type 4 Diabetes Daily Tracking Log

Date		S M T W Th F S		
Meter Readings		**Wellness Index**	**Pain LH Dg Co**	**Meals**
Fasting Glucose		M S-S G VG		Breakfast
Post-breakfast		M S-S G VG		Snack
Other daytime		M S-S G VG		Lunch
Other daytime		M S-S G VG		Dinner
Other daytime		M S-S G VG		Snack
Bedtime		M S-S G VG		Nighttime

Exercise	**Time**	**Type**		**Duration**	**Comments**

Notes

Type 4 Diabetes Daily Tracking Log

Date		S M T W Th F S		
Meter Readings		**Wellness Index**	**Pain LH Dg Co**	**Meals**
Fasting Glucose		M S-S G VG		Breakfast
Post-breakfast		M S-S G VG		Snack
Other daytime		M S-S G VG		Lunch
Other daytime		M S-S G VG		Dinner
Other daytime		M S-S G VG		Snack
Bedtime		M S-S G VG		Nighttime

Exercise	**Time**	**Type**		**Duration**	**Comments**

Notes

Type 4 Diabetes Daily Tracking Log

Date		S M T W Th F S		
Meter Readings		**Wellness Index**	**Pain LH Dg Co**	**Meals**
Fasting Glucose		M S-S G VG		Breakfast
Post-breakfast		M S-S G VG		Snack
Other daytime		M S-S G VG		Lunch
Other daytime		M S-S G VG		Dinner
Other daytime		M S-S G VG		Snack
Bedtime		M S-S G VG		Nighttime

Exercise	**Time**	**Type**		**Duration**	**Comments**

Notes

Type 4 Diabetes Daily Tracking Log

Date		S M T W Th F S				
Meter Readings		**Wellness Index**	**Pain LH Dg Co**	**Meals**		
Fasting Glucose		M S-S G VG		Breakfast		
Post-breakfast		M S-S G VG		Snack		
Other daytime		M S-S G VG		Lunch		
Other daytime		M S-S G VG		Dinner		
Other daytime		M S-S G VG		Snack		
Bedtime		M S-S G VG		Nighttime		

Exercise	**Time**	**Type**		**Duration**	**Comments**

Notes

Type 4 Diabetes Daily Tracking Log

Date		S M T W Th F S				
Meter Readings		**Wellness Index**	**Pain LH Dg Co**	**Meals**		
Fasting Glucose		M S-S G VG		Breakfast		
Post-breakfast		M S-S G VG		Snack		
Other daytime		M S-S G VG		Lunch		
Other daytime		M S-S G VG		Dinner		
Other daytime		M S-S G VG		Snack		
Bedtime		M S-S G VG		Nighttime		

Exercise	**Time**	**Type**		**Duration**	**Comments**

Notes

Type 4 Diabetes Daily Tracking Log

Date		S M T W Th F S				
Meter Readings		**Wellness Index**	**Pain LH Dg Co**	**Meals**		
Fasting Glucose		M S-S G VG		Breakfast		
Post-breakfast		M S-S G VG		Snack		
Other daytime		M S-S G VG		Lunch		
Other daytime		M S-S G VG		Dinner		
Other daytime		M S-S G VG		Snack		
Bedtime		M S-S G VG		Nighttime		

Exercise	**Time**	**Type**		**Duration**	**Comments**

Notes

Index

H

Hall, Gary 56
handheld glucose meters 68
HDL 61, 76
Holmes, Sherlock 154, 155
hyperactive reflex 18, 31
hyperglycemia 4, 164
hypoglycemia 3, 4, 5, 7, 68, 77, 103, 112, 113, 127, 128, 129, 130, 132, 133,
      145, 148, 153, 156, 164, 166, 167, 168, 169, 172

I

Imitrex 41, 45, 49, 123
insulin-producing cells 4
insulin resistance 4, 59, 75, 76, 164
Internet 8, 10

L

LADA 76
lancing 70, 105, 116
Latent Autoimmune Diabetes in Adults 76
LifeScan 69, 70, 99, 104, 105
lightheadedness 18, 26
low blood sugar 9, 16, 18, 68, 103, 113, 114, 129, 132, 133, 145, 153, 156, 168
low glucose 4, 6, 141, 145, 148

M

Medtronic 20, 161
metabolism 3, 6, 72, 73, 74, 78, 97, 100, 133, 134, 154, 156

N

NASA 28
National Diabetes Information Clearinghouse 129
National Dysautonomia Research Foundation 33
National Institute of Diabetes and Digestive and Kidney Diseases 73
National Institutes of Health 60, 73, 141
NDIC 129, 132
NDRF 33
neuro-endocrine 133
Neurocardiogenic 26
neurocardiogenic syncope 26, 31, 32
Neurontin 41, 45, 123, 150
neuropathy 3, 4, 5, 6, 7, 9, 13, 25, 27, 28, 30, 31, 32, 33, 34, 35, 40, 41, 42, 44,

U

UCLA 133, 152
USC 133

V

vasoconstricting 47
vasocontrictor 40, 43

W

Wikipedia 10, 32
www.Type4Diabetes.org 10

Z

Zetia 54

Printed in the United Kingdom
by Lightning Source UK Ltd.
117724UKS00001B/93